The Kaji Review

Emergency Medicine Clinical
Review Book
Volume 1 Part 2

Amy H. Kaji, MD, PhD

Associate Professor of Clinical Medicine
Harbor-UCLA Medical Center
Department of Emergency Medicine

Daniel G. Ostermayer, MD

Assistant Professor of Emergency Medicine
University of Texas Health Science Center at Houston
Department of Emergency Medicine

ASSOCIATE EDITORS

Ami Yamamoto, MD

Harbor-UCLA Medical Center
Department of Emergency Medicine

Kevin P. Beres, DO

University of Texas Health Science Center at Houston
Department of Emergency Medicine

Silas Chiu MD, MS

Harbor-UCLA Medical Center
Department of Emergency Medicine

ASSISTANT EDITOR

Manpreet Singh, MD

Harbor-UCLA Medical Center
Department of Emergency Medicine

SECTION EDITORS

Carrie A. Bakunas, MD
University of Texas Health Science Center at Houston
Department of Emergency Medicine

Elena M. Berry, MD
University of Texas Health Science Center at Houston
Department of Emergency Medicine

Matthew Davey, MD
Oregon Health and Science University
Department of Emergency Medicine

Travis J. Guthrie, MD
University of Texas Health Science Center at Houston
Department of Emergency Medicine

Kathy K. Lee-Ostermayer, MD
Houston Methodist Hospital
Department of Obstetrics and Gynecology

Benjamin Voronin, MD
University of Texas Health Science Center at Houston
Department of Emergency Medicine

Neil Wingkun, MD, MPH
University of Texas Health Science Center at Houston
Department of Emergency Medicine

The Kaji Review

Welcome to the Kaji Review. This book is intended for students, residents, advanced practitioners, and senior physicians alike. Although formatted as a question book, the Kaji Review is really an evidence based clinical case book to advance your bedside knowledge with 774 questions.

We hope you will use this question book to improve clinical care and encourage lifelong learning. Content pulls heavily from textbooks and LLSA readings. Topics are focused on emergency care but also cover outpatient and inpatient medical and surgical topics. Sometimes questions will have more than one correct answer, just like our patients. Don't worry, we will give you a hint on those.

Often the explanations include textbook references, evidence based guidelines, online resources, and specific details of clinical research. If we could find a full text or appropriate video or illustration we included links. Questions are grouped by section so you can focus on specific topics and dive deeply into relevant clinical content.

NEUROLOGY

#1

Treatment for Bell's palsy involves which of the following?

(Choose three answers.)

A. Care to ensure that the cornea remains lubricated with artificial tears, and possibly a patch to cover the affected eye during sleep

B. Glucocorticoids if patient presents within 72 hours

C. Antiviral agents if the paralysis is severe

D. Intravenous fluid hydration

E. None of the above

#1
Answer: A, B, and C

Treatment within 3 days of symptom onset with gluco-corticoids is recommended for all patients with Bell's palsy. The suggested regimen is prednisone (60 to 80 mg/day) for one week. The two largest clinical trials have found no additional benefit for antiviral therapy; however there may be a small subgroup with severe palsy who may have unproven benefit. If an antiviral is to be used, valacyclovir 1000 mg three times a day for one week is appropriate.

- Sullivan FM, et al. Early treatment with prednisolone or acyclovir in Bell's palsy. N Engl J Med. 2007; 357:1598-1607. full text

- Engström M, et al. Prednisolone and valaciclovir in Bell's palsy: a randomised, double-blind, placebo-controlled, multicentre trial. Lancet Neurol. 2008; 7(11): 993-1000. full text

#2

True statements about Myasthenia Gravis (MG) include all of the following, EXCEPT:

A. The muscles most commonly affected include the proximal shoulders.

B. The relative lack of acetylcholine receptors makes these patients relatively resistant to succinylcholine and higher doses must be used to induce paralysis. However, once paralysis is achieved, it may be prolonged.

C. Anticholinesterases are considered first-line agents for treating MG.

D. A major focus of evaluation of MG in the emergency department is ongoing evaluation of the patient's' respiratory status and ability to handle secretions (measure FVC).

E. The diagnosis of MG is confirmed by improved strength in response to a short-acting anticholinesterase agent (Edrophonium test) and by electrophysiologic testing.

#2

Answer: A

The extraocular muscles are most commonly affected in Myasthenia Gravis. Generally symptoms are mild in the morning and progress to episodes of diplopia and ptosis during the day. The facial muscles can also be affected. Patients may report facial fatigue, difficulty chewing, and dysarthria as the the available acetylcholine receptors become saturated. The shoulder girdle muscles are least commonly affected.

- *Rosen's Emergency Medicine - Concepts and Clinical Practice. 8th edition. 2013. Chapter 108: Neuromuscular Disorders. 1443-1444.*

#3

Clinical predictors of traumatic brain injury requiring acute intervention after blunt head trauma in children include all of the following, EXCEPT:

A. Abnormal mental status

B. Clinical signs of skull fracture

C. History of vomiting, scalp hematoma (in children ≤2 years of age)

D. Headache

E. Seizure

#3

Answer: E

Palchak, et al. derived a clinical decision rule for evaluating children with blunt head trauma who were at low risk for traumatic brain injuries (defined by a neurosurgical procedure, antiepileptic medications for more than 1 week, persistent neurologic deficits, or hospitalization for at least 2 nights). Factors associated with traumatic brain injury were:

1. Abnormal mental status
2. Clinical signs of skull fracture
3. History of vomiting
4. Scalp hematoma (in children ≤2 years of age)
5. Headache

These factors identified 97/98 (99%; 95% CI 94% to 100%) of those with traumatic brain injuries on CT scan and 105/105 (100%; 95% CI 97% to 100%) of those with traumatic brain injuries requiring acute intervention.

- *LLSA 2006: Palchak MJ, et al. A decision rule for identifying children at low risk for brain injuries after blunt head trauma. Ann Emerg Med. 2003; 42(4): 492-506. full text*

#4

A 40 year old male presents to you with headache and neck pain after having his neck manipulated by a chiropractor. You suspect a vertebral artery dissection. All of the following are symptoms frequently associated with vertebral artery dissection, EXCEPT:

A. Occipital headache

B. Posterior neck pain

C. Vertebrobasilar ischemic symptoms

D. Unilateral arm pain

E. Urinary retention

#4

Answer: E

The most common presenting complaints of the patient with a vertebral artery dissection is occipital headache and posterior neck pain. The unilateral arm pain that can occur is caused by dissection that involves the vertebral artery within the cervical spine, with local compression on a cervical nerve root, most commonly at the C5-C6 level. The focal ischemic neurologic symptoms are typically those of vertebrobasilar insufficiency.

- *Rosen's Emergency Medicine - Concepts and Clinical Practice. 8th edition. 2013. Chapter 101: Stroke. 1365-1366.*

#5

You are seeing a patient with a third nerve palsy. True statements about the third nerve include all of the following EXCEPT:

    A. The third nerve begins in the midbrain.

    B. The third nerve innervates the superior rectus, inferior rectus, medial rectus, the inferior oblique, and the levator muscles.

    C. Aneurysmal compression of the third nerve typically causes a pupil-sparing third nerve palsy.

    D. If there is a complete, non pupil-sparing third nerve palsy, the patient may have ptosis, a large nonreactive pupil, paralysis of adduction, elevation, and depression.

    E. Partial 3rd nerve palsies may occur, where the pupil may be normal in size or the extra-ocular muscles may only be partially involved.

#5

Answer: C

80-90% of those with an ischemic nerve palsy present with intact pupil function because of the lack of damage to superficial periphery of the 3rd nerve where the majority of the pupillomotor fibers pass. In contrast, aneurysmal compression of superficial pupil fibers very often causes a dilated, unresponsive pupil.

- *Rosen's Emergency Medicine - Concepts and Clinical Practice. 8th edition. 2013. Chapter 71: Ophthalmology. 927-928.*

#6

Which of the following is NOT a treatment option in a patient who presents with a cluster headache?

A. High-flow 100% oxygen

B. Dihydroergotamine (DHE) /Sumatriptan

C. Steroids

D. Verapamil

E. All of the above are treatment options for cluster headache.

#6

Answer: E

High flow 100% oxygen should be administered as initial therapy. DHE and sumatriptan are also effective. However, DHE and sumatriptan should not be used in anyone with cardiovascular risk factors. On discharge, verapamil may be used for prophylaxis, if there are no contraindications. A tapering dose of steroids may also be considered until verapamil can be increased to a therapeutic level (120 mg TID). In practice, most of the abortive and preventive measures are started and titrated by the primary physician.

- *Rosen's Emergency Medicine - Concepts and Clinical Practice. 8th edition. 2013. Chapter 103: Headache Disorders. 1389.*

#7

Regarding internuclear ophthalmoplegia (INO), which of the following is FALSE?

    A. It is characterized by impaired horizontal eye movement with weak adduction of the affected eye and abduction nystagmus of the contralateral eye.

    B. Most patients will recover within a few to several months.

    C. Most cases are due to trauma or infections.

    D. An INO can be confused with a partial third nerve palsy.

    E. The best diagnostic imaging test is an MRI.

#7

Answer: C

Internuclear ophthalmoplegia (INO) is a result of a lesion in the medial longitudinal fasciculus in the dorsomedial brainstem tegmentum of either the pons or the midbrain. It is characterized by impaired horizontal eye movement with weak adduction of the affected eye and abduction nystagmus of the contralateral eye. More than two-thirds of cases result from multiple sclerosis (MS) or cerebrovascular disease. Patients with MS are typically young (less than 45 years old), and the INO is usually bilateral. Patients with cerebrovascular disease are rarely less than 45 years old, have vascular risk factors, and are more likely to have a unilateral INO.

Infections, tumors, and trauma cause most other cases. All patients who present with INO require a brain MRI. Depending on the cause, there can be full recovery or persistent deficits.

- *Cogan DA. Internuclear Ophthalmoplegia, Typical and Atypical. Arch Ophthalmol. 1970; 84(5): 583-589.*

- *Rosen's Emergency Medicine - Concepts and Clinical Practice. 8th edition. 2013. Chapter 21: Diplopia. 181.*

#8

A 19 year old man complains of 1-2 days of lower back pain, lower extremity weakness and tingling, urinary retention and bowel incontinence. Transverse myelitis is in your differential. Which of the following statements is NOT consistent with that disease entity:

A. Progression of symptoms is usually rapid with 2/3 of patient reaching maximal deficit by 24 hours.

B. In addition to motor, sensory and urinary disturbances, patients may complain of back pain and low grade fever.

C. Evaluation is done primarily with emergent MRI to exclude compressive lesions.

D. Steroid treatment should not be delayed as it is the only treatment of known benefit.

E. Transverse myelitis may occur as a complication of syphilis, measles, Lyme disease, and some vaccinations.

#8

Answer: D

The exact cause of transverse myelitis is uncertain. The inflammation that causes such extensive damage to nerve fibers of the spinal cord may result from viral infections, abnormal immune reactions, or insufficient blood flow through the blood vessels located in the spinal cord. Transverse myelitis also may occur as a complication of syphilis, measles, Lyme disease, and some vaccinations, including those for chickenpox and rabies. Treatment with steroids is of unknown benefit. No clinical trials have shown that corticosteroids alter the course of transverse myelitis. Recovery from transverse myelitis usually begins within 2 to 12 weeks of the onset of symptoms and may continue for up to 2 years. However, if there is no improvement within the first 3 to 6 months, significant recovery is unlikely.

- *Rosen's Emergency Medicine - Concepts and Clinical Practice. 8th edition. 2013. Chapter 106: Spinal Cord Disorders. 1424.*

#9

Which of the following is not part of the classic tetrad of findings in Neuroleptic Malignant Syndrome (NMS)?

A. Renal failure

B. Altered mental status

C. Rigidity

D. Autonomic dysfunction

E. Hyperthermia

#9

Answer: A

NMS consists of a tetrad of findings:

1. Changes in mental status
2. Extrapyramidal symptoms
3. Hyperpyrexia
4. Autonomic instability

The findings are not always present, with the most common being extrapyramidal symptoms and hyperpyrexia. The catatonic signs are described as "lead pipe rigidity," and patient's temperature often ranges between 38-40 ºC.   Patients may demonstrate an agitated delirium or encephalopathy, making the diagnosis difficult to distinguish from an infectious meningitis or encephalitis if there are not extrapyramidal symptoms present. The autonomic instability usually manifests with tachycardia, but patients can also have labile blood pressures.

- *Rosen's Emergency Medicine - Concepts and Clinical Practice. 8th edition. 2013. Chapter 161: Antipsychotics. 2049.*

#10

Regarding spinal epidural abscess, which of the following statements is FALSE:

A. Major risk factors include diabetes, chronic renal failure, alcoholism, immunosuppression and IV drug abuse.

B. Infection is most frequently identified as a skin and soft tissue source that is usually confined to the adipose tissue of the dorsal epidural space where there is a rich venous plexus.

C. CT is the imaging modality of choice and needs to be obtained emergently.

D. ESR is not specific for this disease entity but is almost always elevated.

E. Staph aureus is the most common organism, cultured in over 50% of cases.

#10

Answer: C

The imaging modality of choice is MRI. Staphylococcus aureus is the most prevalent organism cultured in more than 50% of cases. Other frequently identified organisms include aerobic and anaerobic strep, E. coli, and Pseudomonas aeruginosa.

- *Rosen's Emergency Medicine - Concepts and Clinical Practice. 8th edition. 2013. Chapter 106: Spinal Cord Disorders. 1426.*

#11

A 45 year old male with a long history of alcohol abuse presents with new-onset wrist drop. He denies any trauma to his arm nor any previous episodes. Characteristics of a radial nerve palsy due to lesion in the middle third of the arm include all of the following EXCEPT:

(Choose two answers.)

A. Paralysis of all extensors of the wrist.

B. Paralysis of all extensors of the digits

C. Paralysis of all forearm supinators

D. Numbness over the dorsoradial aspect of the hand and the dorsal aspect of the radial 3 and ½ digits.

E. Numbness over the distal and lateral forearm.

#11
Answer: C and E

Radial nerve palsy in the middle third of the arm is characterized by palsy or paralysis of all extensors of the wrist and digits. The biceps brachii, which is innervated by the musculocutaneous nerve, also supinates the forearm; therefore, not all supination will be compromised. Very proximal lesions may also affect the triceps.

Numbness occurs on the dorsoradial aspect of the hand and the dorsal aspect of the radial 3 ½ digits. Sensation over the distal and lateral forearm is supplied by the lateral antebrachial cutaneous nerve, and therefore is preserved. Sensation over the distal and lateral forearm is supplied by the lateral antebrachial cutaneous nerve, and therefore is preserved. If entrapment of the radial nerve in the arm is suspected, obtain radiographs to rule out a fracture, healing callus, or tumor as the cause of entrapment.

- *Rosen's Emergency Medicine - Concepts and Clinical Practice. 8th edition. 2013. Chapter 107: Peripheral Nerve Disorders. 1433-1434.*

#12

A 45 year old male presents to the ED after he sustains some mild head trauma while attempting to flee from law enforcement. There was apparently a brief episode of loss of consciousness without vomiting, and the patient is brought by police officers who would like medical clearance to custody. Which of the following features is LEAST consistent with a concussion?

    A. Anterograde and retrograde amnesia lasting 4-5 hours

    B. Mild/moderate headache

    C. Inability to recall his name and date of birth

    D. Seizure on impact

    E. Signs of trauma to the scalp

#12

Answer: C

Concussion is an injury to the brain that results in temporary loss of normal brain function. It usually is caused by a blow to the head. In many cases, there are no external signs of head trauma. A concussion does not require loss of consciousness. Degree of concussive symptoms correlate with severity of injury. Patients may have anterograde and retrograde amnesia, where the retrograde amnesia is of greater severity than the anterograde symptoms. In this case, the patient cannot recall autobiographical information. This is not consistent with concussive symptoms and suggests hysteria or malingering.

- *Ropper AH, et al. Concussion. New Engl J Med. 2007; 356(2): 166-172.*

#13

You are seeing a patient with what you believe is an isolated third nerve palsy. Which of the following features may DECREASE your concern for an intracranial aneurysm as the cause?

A. The pupil appears to be fixed and dilated.

B. The pupil is dilated and very sluggishly reactive.

C. The patient complains of the worst headache of his life.

D. The pupil is uninvolved – it reacts normally to light.

E. There is an isolated third nerve palsy and the patient has a strong family of SAH.

#13

Answer: D

A neurologically isolated third nerve palsy with a normal pupillary sphincter and completely palsied extraocular muscles (complete external dysfunction) is almost never caused by an aneurysm, although there are case reports that describe this phenomenon in the setting of a basilar artery aneurysm. Pupil-involving third nerve palsy should be assumed to be due to aneurysmal compression until proven otherwise. Patients should undergo MRI and MRA (or CTA) to exclude an aneurysm. The differential should also include orbital fracture, malignancies, and diabetic neuropathies.

- *Keane JR. Aneurysms and third nerve palsies. Ann Neurol. 1983; 14(6): 696-7.*

- *Lustbader JM, et al. Painless, pupil-sparing but otherwise complete oculomotor nerve paresis caused by basilar artery aneurysm. Case report. Arch Ophthalmol. 1988 May; 106(5): 583-4.*

#14

In which of the following types of seizure presentations is a metabolic etiology most likely?

A. Generalized tonic-clonic

B. Simple partial

C. Complex partial

D. Myoclonic with altered mental status

E. Absence

#14

Answer: D

Patients with myoclonus and altered consciousness are more likely to have a metabolic cause of the seizure. Uremic and hepatic encephalopathy are common causes of myoclonic seizures, although electrolyte disturbances and hypoglycemia can also cause myoclonic seizures, as well.

The common forms of status epilepticus are:

1. **Simple partial** — characterized by continuous or repeated focal motor seizures, focal sensory symptoms, or cognitive symptoms (eg, aphasia) without impaired consciousness.

2. **Complex partial** — characterized by continuous or repeated episodes of focal motor, sensory, or cognitive symptoms with impaired consciousness.

3. **Generalized tonic-clonic** — always associated with impaired consciousness.

4. **Absence** - characterized by altered consciousness but not unconsciousness.

5. **Myoclonic** - characterized by frequent myoclonic jerks, usually in the setting of altered mental status.

6. **Tonic-clonic** - seizures may be the initial manifestation of status epilepticus, or may represent secondary generalization from other seizure types.

- *Rosen's Emergency Medicine - Concepts and Clinical Practice. 8th edition. 2013. Chapter 18: Seizures. 156-161.*

#15

Which of the following is FALSE regarding the anti-epileptic agent, Levetiracetam (Keppra)?

    A. It is primarily metabolized by the liver.

    B. It does not cause hypotension.

    C. It does not cause cardiovascular depression.

    D. It does not require drug level monitoring.

    E. It comes in both an IV and oral formulation.

#15

Answer: A

Nau KM, et al. retrospectively analyzed the use, safety, and efficacy of levetiracetam in ICU patients. The drug does not undergo hepatic metabolism, does not require serum level monitoring and has a hemodynamically stable profile. Traditional antiepileptics such as phenytoin have the potential for cardiovascular depression and hypotension.

- *Nau KM, et al. Safety and Efficacy of Levetiracetam for Critically Ill Patients with Seizures. Neurocritical Care. 2009; 11(1): 34-7.*

#16

A patient presents with a headache, and you are considering a diagnosis of migraine. Which of the following is part of the POUNDing mnemonic to help distinguish migraines from other primary headache disorders?

A. Is it a pulsating headache?

B. Does it last between 4 and 72 hours without medication?

C. Is it unilateral?

D. Is there nausea?

E. Is the headache debilitating?

F. All of the above

#16

Answer: F

Detsky, et al. assessed two questions in a systematic review to guide clinicians in evaluating patients with headaches.

1. Is this headache a migraine?
2. Does this patient require neuroimaging?

The 5 questions for determining if a patient's headache could be a migraine are:

1. Is the headache **P**ulsating?
2. Is the headache duration of 4-72 h**O**urs?
3. Is the headache **U**nilateral?
4. Is the headache associated with **N**ausea?
5. Is the headache **D**isabling to daily activity?

If the patient answers "yes" to 4 or more of the 5 questions, the positive likelihood ratio is 24 (95% CI 1.5 -388) for a migraine. For 3 criteria, the LR is 3.5 (95%CI 1.3-9.2); and for 1 or 2 criteria, the LR is 0.41 (95%CI 0.32-0.52).

- *Rosen's Emergency Medicine - Concepts and Clinical Practice. 8th edition. 2013. Chapter 103: Headache Disorders. 1386-1387.*

- *Detsky ME, et al. Does this patient with headache have a migraine or need neuroimaging? JAMA. 2006; 296(10): 1274-83. full text*

#17

Which of the following is NOT predictive of CVA after a patient presents with a TIA?

A. Unilateral numbness

B. Age

C. Symptom duration

D. Unilateral weakness

E. Speech impairment

#17
Answer: A

The derived and validated risk stratification scores for TIA are:

California

1. Age > 60 y
2. Diabetes
3. Transient ischemic attack duration > 10 min
4. Weakness with transient ischemic attack
5. Speech impairment with transient ischemic attack

ABCD

1. Age > 60 y
2. Blood pressure (initial systolic blood pressure > 140 mm Hg or diastolic blood pressure > 90 mm Hg)
3. Clinical feature: unilateral weakness
4. Clinical feature: speech disturbance without weakness
5. Duration of symptoms 10–60 min
6. Duration of symptoms > 60 min

ABCD2

1. Age > 60 y
2. Blood pressure (systolic blood pressure > 140 mm Hg or diastolic blood pressure > 90 mm Hg)
3. Clinical feature: unilateral weakness
4. Clinical feature: speech disturbance without weakness Duration of symptoms 10-60 min
5. Duration of symptoms > 60 min
6. Diabetes

Johnston, et al. derived the California score from a cohort of 1,707 patients treated by emergency physicians and given a diagnosis of transient ischemic attack. The five variables found to be independently predictive of stroke: age older than 60 years (odds ratio [OR] 1.8), diabetes (OR 2.0), symptom duration greater than 10 minutes (OR 2.3), and symptoms of weakness (OR 1.9) or speech impairment (either dysarthria or aphasia) (OR 1.5).

In patients with no risk factors, there were no strokes at 90 days; for patients with all 5 risk factors, 34% experienced a stroke. Roughly half of strokes occurred within the first 48 hours after presentation.

- *Cucciara B, et al. Transient Ischemic Attack: Risk Stratification and Treatment. Ann Emerg Med. 2008; 52: S27-S39. full text*

- *MDCalc - ABCD2 http://www.mdcalc.com/abcd2-score-for-tia/*

#18

You have just performed a traumatic lumbar puncture on an individual and are having difficulty interpreting the results because of the large number of RBCs. There are 50 WBCs in the CSF, but there are 2500 RBCs in the CSF. The best way to correct the WBCs for the RBCs is to:

A. Subtract one WBC for every 250 RBC.

B. Subtract one WBC for every 500 RBC.

C. Calculate the predicted CSF WBC count from the formula: predicted CSF WBC= CSF RBC x (peripheral blood WBC/ peripheral blood RBC)

D. If you can read through the container, there is no meningitis.

E. Repeat the lumbar puncture.

#18

Answer: C

Accidental trauma during an LP from puncturing a venule will increase the number of both RBCs and WBCs in the CSF. If the peripheral WBC count is not abnormally low or high, a commonly used method is to subtract one WBC for every 500 to 1500 RBCs if a traumatic tap is suspected. However this still provides a vague estimate of the WBC count. The presence or absence of otherwise unexplained xanthochromia also may help distinguish a traumatic tap from subarachnoid hemorrhage as long as the LP is performed at least six hours after the onset of headache. A more accurate method is to calculate the predicted CSF WBC count with the the following formula:

Predicted CSF WBC count/microL = CSF RBC count x (peripheral blood WBC count ÷ peripheral blood RBC count)

Mayefsky, et al. in a study of 720 reported traumatic LPs found that a CSF WBC count that was more than 10 times the predicted value had a 48% positive predictive value for bacterial meningitis, while a value less than 10 times the predicted value had a 99% negative predictive value for meningitis.

Perry et al, recently concluded in a study of 1739 patients being ruled out for subarachnoid hemorrhage in 12 Canadian EDs that fewer than 2000×10^6/L red blood cells on LP in addition to no xanthochromia excluded the diagnosis of aneurysmal subarachnoid hemorrhage, with a sensitivity of 100% (95% confidence interval 74.7% to 100%) and specificity of 91.2% (88.6% to 93.3%).

- Edlow JA, Caplan LR. Avoiding pitfalls in the diagnosis of subarachnoid hemorrhage. N Engl J Med. 2000; 342(1): 29–36. full text

- Mayefsky JH, Roghmann KJ. Determination of leukocytosis in trau-

matic spinal tap specimens. Am J Med. 1987 Jun; 82(6): 1175-81.

. *Peds EM Morsels http://pedemmorsels.com/traumatic-lumbar-puncture/*

. *Perry JJ, et al. Differentiation between traumatic tap and aneurysmal subarachnoid hemorrhage: prospective cohort study. BMJ. 2015 Feb 18; 350:h568. full text*

#19

**In terms of acute treatment in the ED for those present-
ing with a CVA, which of the following is NOT recommended?**

    A. Permissive hypertension

    B. Reverse trendelenburg

    C. Intravenous fluid administration

    D. Keep the head of the bed flat

    E. None of the above

#19

Answer: B

Initial treatment of patients with transient ischemic attack should begin with basic supportive care measures to optimize potentially compromised cerebral blood flow. This includes positioning the patient with the head of the bed flat, permissive hypertension, and administration of intravenous fluids. Head position at 0 degrees may preserve cerebral perfusion pressure, and the choice of head position may have the greatest importance in patients with large vessel occlusions. Studies using transcranial doppler monitoring have shown that mean flow velocity in the middle cerebral artery can increase 20% when head position is lowered from 30 degrees to 0 degrees.

Permissive hypertension involves avoiding aggressive blood pressure normalization in the setting of a CVA. Cerebral perfusion, particularly in regions dependent on collateral blood flow, may be directly dependent on systemic blood pressure. A controlled trial of nimodipine in acute ischemic stroke demonstrated poorer outcomes with blood pressure lowering. Additional studies have also identified early blood pressure lowering as a predictor of poor outcomes after stroke. Isotonic intravenous fluids should be given to ensure euvolemia and maintain intravascular volume, since hypotension in the setting of a CVA portends poor neurologic recovery.

- *Cucciara B, et al. Transient Ischemic Attack: Risk Stratification and Treatment. Ann Emerg Med. 2008; 52: S27-S39. full text*

#20

Which of the following is INCORRECT regarding cerebral vascular accident (CVA) prevention after a patient presents with a transient ischemic attack (TIA)?

A. Once hemorrhage is excluded by imaging, an antiplatelet agent is indicated.

B. Anticoagulation with warfarin has been found to be beneficial in the immediate peri-TIA presentation.

C. If the patient has >70% carotid stenosis and is symptomatic, a carotid endarterectomy is indicated.

D. If the patient is found to have infective endocarditis, then antibiotics and cardiology consultation are indicated.

E. If the patient also has atrial fibrillation which is thought to be the etiology of the TIA, then warfarin treatment has been found to be more effective in preventing recurrent stroke when compared to aspirin therapy.

#20

Answer: B

Regarding carotid endarterectomy and revasculariza-tion, 2 large randomized trials, the European Carotid Surgery Trial and the North American Symptomatic Carotid Endarterectomy Trial demonstrated a 10-15% decrease in recurrent CVA if the patient with a > 70% carotid stenosis underwent endarterectomy.

Warfarin therapy should be reserved for patients who have a recurrent CVA or CVA due to atrial fibrillation. In a meta-analysis of 12 trials involving almost 13,000 patients with recurrent CVA , warfarin was associated with a 39% relative risk reduction (95% CI 22% to 52%) compared with antiplatelet therapy. In patients with ischemic stroke without atrial fibrillation, no benefit has been shown regarding anticoagulation when compared with aspirin. Therapy should be individualized to patients who are at risk for falls and head trauma due to the bleeding risk associated with systemic anticoagulation.

Embolic TIA/CVA caused by bacterial endocarditis requires immediate antibiotics, cardiology and cardiothoracic consultation. There is a high risk of hemorrhagic conversion in these patients, and IV anticoagulation should not be started.

Overall, in patients with stroke or transient ischemic attack, long-term aspirin therapy reduces the risk of recurrent stroke, myocardial infarction, or vascular death by about 20%. Aspirin and extended-release dipyridamole have shown greater efficacy in preventing recurrent stroke in patients with severe cerebrovascular disease. The Clopidogrel for High Atherothrombotic Risk and Ischemic Stabilization, Management, and Avoidance study, did not demonstrate an overall benefit to combination of aspirin and clopidogrel therapy.

- *Cucciara B, et al. Transient Ischemic Attack: Risk Stratification and Treatment. Ann Emerg Med. 2008; 52: S27-S39. full text*

- *Bhatt DL, et al. Clopidogrel and aspirin versus aspirin alone for the prevention of atherothrombotic events. N Engl J Med. 2006; 354:1706-1717. full text*

- *Rothwell PM, et al. Endarterectomy for symptomatic carotid stenosis in relation to clinical subgroups and timing of surgery. Lancet. 2004; 363:915-924*

#21

Regarding the initiation of anti-platelet therapy for patients with TIA, which of the following is NOT recommended by the AHA/American Stroke Association and the American College of Chest Physicians as long-term therapy?

 A. Aspirin 50mg to 325 mg per day

 B. Aspirin 25 mg plus extended-release dipyridamole 200 mg twice a day

 C. Clopidogrel 75 mg per day

 D. Aspirin and clopidogrel combined

#21

Answer: D

The American Heart Association/American Stroke Association (AHA/ASA) and American College of Chest Physicians (ACCP) recommend use of antiplatelet therapy for patients with noncardioembolic transient ischemic attack.

Long term preventative therapy options:

- Aspirin 50 to 325 mg/day
- Combination of aspirin 325 mg and extended-release dipyridamole 200 mg twice daily
- Clopidogrel 75 mg/day

All of the above options are acceptable, and therapy should be individualized for the patient's risk. If clopidogrel is prescribed, it should be given as a single agent, and not in combination with aspirin, unless there is acute coronary syndrome or recent stenting.

In 2006 and 2011, the guideline read, "The addition of aspirin to clopidogrel increases the risk of hemorrhage and is not recommended for routine secondary prevention after ischemic stroke or TIA (Class III; Level of Evidence A)."

In 2014, the caveat that combination aspirin and clopidogrel may be beneficial for patients with acute coronary syndromes or recent vascular stenting was added with the recommendation: "The combination of aspirin and clopidogrel might be considered for initiation within 24 hours of a minor ischemic stroke or TIA and for continuation for 21 days (Class IIb; Level of Evidence B)." Still, "the combination of aspirin and clopidogrel, when initiated days to years after a minor stroke or TIA and continued for 2 to 3 years, increases the risk of hemorrhage relative to either agent alone and is not recommended for routine long-term secondary prevention after ischemic stroke or TIA (Class III; Level of Evidence A)."

- *Cucciara B, et al. Transient Ischemic Attack: Risk Stratification and Treatment. Ann Emerg Med. 2008; 52: S27-S39. full text*

- *Kernan WN, et al. Guidelines for the prevention of stroke in patients with stroke and transient ischemic attack: a guideline for healthcare professionals from the American Heart Association/American Stroke Association. Stroke. 2014 Jul; 45(7): 2160-236. full text*

- *Furie KL, et al. Guidelines for the prevention of stroke in patients with stroke or transient ischemic attack: a guideline for healthcare professionals from the american heart association/american stroke association. Stroke. 2011 Jan; 42(1): 227-76. full text*

- *Sacco RL, et al. Guidelines for prevention of stroke in patients with ischemic stroke or transient ischemic attack: a statement for healthcare professionals from the American Heart Association/American Stroke Association Council on Stroke: co-sponsored by the Council on Cardiovascular Radiology and Intervention: the American Academy of Neurology affirms the value of this guideline. Stroke. 2006; 37: 577-617 full text*

- *Albers GW, et al. Antithrombotic and thrombolytic therapy for ischemic stroke: the Seventh ACCP Conference on Antithrombotic and Thrombolytic Therapy. Chest. 2004; 126: 483S-512S. full text*

#22

You are examining a patient who has 250 WBCs in the CSF, a glucose that is 35 (low), and a protein that is 150, with a negative gram stain. Historical and physical exam features that may be consistent with an aseptic meningitis include which of the following?

    A. Exposure to rodents

    B. Exposure to ticks

    C. Exposure to high-risk sexual activity

    D. Physical exam findings consistent with mumps

    E. Exposure to drugs

    F. All of the above

#22
Answer: F

Aseptic meningitis is caused by both viruses and other atypical infections such as zoonotics. Physical findings in aseptic meningitis are similar to bacterial meningitis except fever is generally more mild. Neurologic features can include cranial nerve palsies involving the facial nerve, and even bilateral (more common in Lyme Meningitis).

Lymphocytic choriomeningitis virus (LCMV), a human zoonosis caused by a rodent-borne arenavirus, is found in the urine and feces of rodents, and is transmitted to by direct contact.

Other tick-borne diseases that cause aseptic meningitis include Rocky Mountain Spotted Fever and Ehrlichiosis. Also consider fungal infections (Cryptococcosis and Coccidioidomycosis) in the differentials, especially in patients who are immunocompromised. High-risk sexual activity predisposes patients to HIV, Herpes meningitis, and Syphilitic meningitis. Mumps virus can cause aseptic meningitis as well.

Although drug-induced meningitis is a diagnosis of exclusion, NSAIDS, antibiotics, and immunosuppressants and IVIG have all been implicated. The medication likely causes direct meningeal irritation and inflammation, although the mechanism may be different for each class of medication.

- *Lee BE, Davies HD. Aseptic Meningitis. Current Opinion in Internal Medicine. 2007; 6(4): 370-375.*

- *Jolles S, et al. Drug-induced aseptic meningitis: diagnosis and management. Drug Saf. 2000; 22(3): 215-226.*

#23

You are seeing a 28 year old female with a history of Myasthenia Gravis. She presents with generalized weakness, dyspnea that is worse with being supine, as well as bulbar symptoms, such as dysphagia. You are concerned that she may have myasthenic crisis. TRUE statements about this entity include which of the following?

(Choose three answers.)

A. Myasthenic crisis may be precipitated by a variety of factors including infection, surgery, or tapering of immunosuppression.

B. A number of medications can increase the weakness in myasthenia as well as precipitate a crisis.

C. Intubation should only be considered when vital capacity (VC) gets to < 5 ml/kg

D. Intubation should be considered when the maximal inspiratory force (MIF) is -70 cm H_2O

E. Plasmapheresis or IVIG should be considered for therapy.

#23

Answer: A, B, and E

Intubation should be considered if serial measurements of the VC show values less than 20 mL/kg or if the NIF is worse than -30 cm H20. Plasmapheresis (plasma exchange) may offer the greatest benefit by removing the acetylcholine receptor antibodies from the body. Multiple rounds of plasmapheresis are usually required. IVIG will also help reverse the crisis since the pooled immunoglobulins can bind the acetylcholine receptor antibodies. Many medications, such as beta blockers and antibiotics, can precipitate a myasthenic crisis, as can changes in immunosuppressives or recent infection or surgery.

- *Rosen's Emergency Medicine - Concepts and Clinical Practice. 8th edition. 2013. Chapter 108: Neuromuscular Disorders. 1443-1444.*

#24

You are seeing a patient that appears to have a stroke. The neurology resident states he believes your patient has Wallenberg's syndrome, which is due to lateral medullary infarction (vertebral artery involvement). Which of the following signs and/or symptoms are not consistent with Wallenberg's?

A. Complete bilateral horizontal gaze palsy

B. Nystagmus

C. Difficulty sitting upright without support

D. Loss of pain or temperature sensation in the ipsilateral face and contralateral limb and trunk

#24

Answer: A

Crossed findings in examination of a patient with ipsilateral face and contralateral body should always prompt concern for a brain stem or medullary infarct.

Lateral medullary infarction (Wallenberg syndrome) is caused by vertebral artery occlusion, with sensory deficits affecting the trunk and extremities on the opposite side of the infarction and sensory deficits affecting the face and cranial nerves on the same side of the infarct. The infarct damages:

1. The spinothalamic tract resulting in loss of pain and temperature sensation on the opposite side of the body.
2. The cerebellum or the inferior cerebellar peduncle causing ataxia.
3. The hypothalamospinal fibers causing damage to the sympathetic relay producing a Horner syndrome.

Physical exam may reveal:

1. Difficulty sitting upright without support due to cerebellar infarction. Patients often feel as if they are being pulled to the side of the lesion
2. Hypotonia of the ipsilateral arm
3. Blurred vision or diplopia
4. Nystagmus, often with both horizontal and vertical rotary components
5. Limb ataxia
6. Sensory symptoms with loss of pain and temperature on the opposite side of the contralateral limb and ipsilateral face

The incorrect answer, "complete bilateral horizontal

gaze palsy" would be a symptom consistent with BASI-LAR artery occlusion, and not the VERTEBRAL artery. Oculomotor symptoms and signs are common with symptomatic BASILAR artery occlusion, and can include:

1. Complete bilateral horizontal gaze palsy
2. Unilateral horizontal conjugate gaze palsy
3. Unilateral or bilateral internuclear ophthalmoplegia (INO)
4. One-and-a-half syndrome (a conjugate gaze palsy combined with an INO).

• *Schneider JI, Olshaker JS. Vertigo, vertebrobasilar disease, and posterior circulation ischemic stroke. Emerg Med Clin North Am. 2012; 30(3): 681-93. full text*

#25

You are seeing a patient who has Bell's palsy. She asks you about her prognosis. Which of the following factors affect prognosis for recovery?

(Choose three answers.)

    A. Severity of the facial weakness

    B. If some recovery is seen within the first 21 days

    C. Whether it is idiopathic or due to Herpes Zoster

    D. Age

    E. Season when affected

#25

Answer: A, B and C

The prognosis of Bell's palsy is related to the severity of the lesion. There is a 94% rate of return to normal facial nerve function if the lesion is incomplete. Rate of return for complete lesions is reported at approximately 60%. When compared with herpes zoster viral infection, an idiopathic palsy is associated with a worse prognosis. The sooner the signs of recovery (especially if within 3 weeks), the greater the chance for complete return of normal function.

- Peitersen E. *The natural history of Bell's palsy. Am J Otol. 1982; 4(2): 107-11.*

#26

You are doing the Hallpike test (Dix-Hallpike, Nylan-Barany) test on a patient that presents with vertigo. TRUE statements about this include which of the following?

(Choose two answers.)

A. This test diagnoses otoliths in the anterior semi-circular canal.

B. The patient should have his/her eyes closed throughout the test.

C. If the test is positive, the patient will develop reproduction of his symptoms and usually nystagmus.

D. If the side that you tested is positive, then you can treat the patient with the Epley maneuver.

E. The head should not overhang the edge of the gurney when he lies down.

#26

Answer: C and D

The Hallpike test diagnoses otoliths in the POSTERIOR semicircular canal, which is oriented 45 degrees from the vertical. The patient should be sitting upright in the gurney and positioned far enough back so when laying down, the head overhangs the edge of the gurney. The patient should be instructed to keep eyes open as it is extremely important to document the presence and direction of nystagmus. The change in position should happen quickly over 2 seconds from sitting to lying. If otoliths are present, there is usually a few seconds delay of no symptoms followed by reproduction of the vertigo with nystagmus towards the involved side. If the side tested is positive, then the patient can be treated with the Epley maneuver.

- *Hallpike CS and Dix MR. The pathology symptomatology and diagnosis of certain common disorders of the vestibular system. Proc R Soc Med. 1952 Jun;45(6):341-54. full text*

#27

Regarding subarachnoid hemorrhage (SAH), which of the following statements is TRUE?

(Choose two answers.)

A. The most common cause of SAH is aneurysm rupture.

B. 1/100 headaches presenting to the ED will have a SAH.

C. Most aneurysms occur in the posterior circulation.

D. The Hunt and Hess score has poor interobserver agreement.

E. Post-menopausal women are more commonly affected by SAH than men.

#27

Answer: D and E

Trauma is the leading cause of SAH, not aneurysmal rupture. Intracranial aneurysms are more commonly in the arteries of the Circle of Willis, but can also occur in other branches. Based on autopsy data, the rate of aneurysms is 0.4–3.6% of all individuals. The majority of aneurysms occur in the anterior circulation.

Scoring systems for assessing the patient's clinical status are the Hunt and Hess grading system and the World Federation of Neurosurgical Societies (WFNS) scale. Hunt and Hess' original article correlated clinical grade with mortality, although the score has low interobserver agreement. The incidence of SAH is more common in Blacks and Hispanics than Whites. Post-menopausal women are more affected than men.

Scales for Clinical Rating of Subarachnoid Hemorrhage Patients

World Federation of Neurosurgical Societies (WFNS) SAH grade		
WFNS Grade	Glasgow Coma Score	Major Focal Deficit
0 (unruptured)	—	—
1	15	Absent
2	13–14	Absent
3	13–14	Present
4	7–12	Present/absent
5	3–6	Present/absent

Hunt and Hess Scale	
Grade	Description
0	Unruptured
1	Asymptomatic, or mild headache and slight nuchal rigidity
2	Moderate to severe headache, nuchal rigidity, no neurologic deficit other than a cranial nerve palsy
3	Mild focal deficit, lethargy, or confusion
4	Stupor, moderate to severe hemiparesis, or dearly decerebrate rigidity
5	Deep coma, decerebrate rigidity, moribund appearance
Add one grade for serious systemic disease (e.g., HTN, DM, severe atherosclerosis, COPD) or severe vasospasm on arteriography	

- *Edlow JA, et al. Aneurysmal subarachnoid hemorrhage: Update for emergency physicians. J Emerg Med. 2008 Apr; 34(3): 237-51. full text*

- *Degen LA, et al. Interobserver variability of grading scales for aneurysmal subarachnoid hemorrhage. Stroke. 2011 Jun; 42(6): 1546-9. full text*

#28

Regarding SAH, which of the following are pitfalls leading to misdiagnosis?

    A. Failing to pursue the diagnosis because pain medications eased the symptoms

    B. Failure to recognize that xanthochromia may be absent very early (< 12 h) and very late (> 2 weeks)

    C. Not realizing that the sensitivity of CT scan diminishes with time of onset of symptoms

    D. Failure to realize that CT scan can be falsely negative in a patient with a hematocrit < 30%

    E. All of the above

#28
Answer: E

Reasons for Misdiagnosis	Points of Caution
Failure to know the spectrum of presentations of subarachnoid hemorrhage	**Only 10% of severe quick onset** headaches are from SAH. Patients can also have **meningismus, nausea, or vomiting accompanying** the headache.
Not thoroughly evaluating patients with frequent headaches	Most headaches are the worst of their life or clearly different than their usual headache.
Is the onset abrupt?	The onset of headaches are usually sudden.
Is the quality and severity different from prior headaches?	All headaches should be compared to the patient's normal quality and severity.
Failure to appreciate that the headache can improve spontaneously or with non-narcotic analgesics	A SAH may improve with non-narcotic analgesic. History and physical should dictate decision making.
Failure to understand the limitations of computed tomography (CT) scans	**In patients scanned within 6 h of headache onset, the CT scan may be 92-100% sensitive.** CT scan can be falsely negative for blood at hematocrit level of < 30%.
CT scans are less sensitive with increasing time from onset of headache	**By 3 and 7 days after the bleed,** the sensitivity of CT falls to **85% and 50%,** respectively.
CT scan can be falsely negative with small volume bleeds (spectrum bias)	**In patients with small sentinel** bleeds, the CT scan **is less likely to show blood.** In differing clinical settings, the diagnostic accuracy of a test will vary.
Failure to understand the limitations of xanthochromia measurement	**Xanthochromia may be absent** very early (< 12 h) and very late (> 2 weeks).

- *Edlow JA, et al. Aneurysmal Subarachnoid Hemorrhage: Update for Emergency Physicians. J Emerg Med. 2008 Apr; 34(3): 237-51. full text*

#29

Limitations with CT for diagnosis of SAH include which of the following?

A. The accuracy of CT is less in the acute period.

B. Studies regarding the utility of CT are subject to "spectrum bias."

C. Both of the above

D. Neither of the above

#29

Answer: B

Perry, et al. demonstrated that among 953 patients scanned within 6 hours of headache onset, all 121 patients with subarachnoid hemorrhage were identified, demonstrating a sensitivity of 100% (95% CI, 97.0% - 100.0%), specificity of 100% (95 CI 99.5% - 100%). The sensitivity of CT scan is greatest in the acute period and decreases after 6 hours.

The most underappreciated limitation of CT is "spectrum bias." Spectrum bias is the variation in the performance of a diagnostic test due to the setting and mix of patients. Unless the study population is identical to patients being treated in your emergency department, the performance of the test may differ. Specifically regarding CT scans, various radiologists will have differing expertise (sensitivity and specificity) in their interpretations.

Until multiple studies confirm 100% sensitivity of ultra-early CT scanning in SAH, all patients being evaluated for SAH whose CT scans are normal should be further evaluated with a lumbar puncture.

- Edlow JA, et al. Aneurysmal Subarachnoid Hemorrhage: Update for Emergency Physicians. J Emerg Med. 2008; 34: 237-251. full text

#30

Regarding SAH and LPs, which of the following is TRUE?

    A. Traumatic taps occur 10-15% of the time.

    B. Visual inspection is more sensitive than spectro-photometry for detection of xanthochromia.

    C. Both of the above

    D. Neither of the above.

#30

Answer: A

Cerebrospinal fluid (CSF) analysis also has limitations, and no methods is perfect at distinguishing traumatic taps from SAH. Traumatic taps are estimated to occur 10-15% of the time. Xanthochromia is the yellowish hue of the CSF that results from hemoglobin breakdown into oxyhemoglobin, methemoglobin, and bilirubin. Xanthochromia by lab spectrophotometry can take 12 h to detect, but to the naked eye, it may be visible earlier. Spectrophotometry detection of xanthochromia is more sensitive, however.

- *Edlow JA, et al. Aneurysmal Subarachnoid Hemorrhage: Update for Emergency Physicians. J Emerg Med. 2008 Apr; 34(3): 237-51. full text*

#31

Does a patient presenting with a severe headache, normal neurologic exam, normal CT, and normal CSF analysis require further evaluation for a subarachnoid hemorrhage with an angiogram?

    A. Yes

    B. No

#31

Answer: B

The vast majority of the patient described above, with normal neuro exam, normal CT and normal LP have excellent outcomes. Wijdicks, et al. in a retrospective study of 71 patients described in the question, had no SAH diagnosed at 3.3 years of follow-up. Prospective studies have also confirmed this finding.

- *Edlow JA, et al. Aneurysmal Subarachnoid Hemorrhage: Update for Emergency Physicians. J Emerg Med. 2008 Apr; 34(3): 237-51. full text*

#32

True or False: An LP-first strategy (no CT) for SAH is evidence-based and should be the standard of care?

    A. True

    B. False

#32

Answer: B

A LP-first strategy may be safe in patients without signs of elevated ICP or neurologic deficits, but it is not an evidence based approach. The current standard of care, which includes a CT scan followed by an LP, is well supported by the medical literature. Proponents of an LP-first strategy argue that it will prevent clinicians from avoiding performing the LP. The greatest concern with this approach is the risk of herniation.

- *Edlow JA, et al. Aneurysmal Subarachnoid Hemorrhage: Update for Emergency Physicians. J Emerg Med. 2008 Apr; 34(3): 237-51. full text*

#33

True or False: A CT-angiogram strategy for diagnosis of SAH would likely lead to fewer neurosurgical work-ups and overall decreased administration of contrast material.

    A. True

    B. False

#33
Answer: B

Many clinicians in sites with current generation CT scanners may favor a CTA first approach to diagnosing SAH. Carstairs, et al. in a study of 116 patients being ruled out for subarachnoid hemorrhage, found 5.1% to have aneurysms on CTA with a normal non-con CT but positive CSF findings. Three patients had a positive CTA with normal CT and normal CSF, but these patients most likely had asymptomatic aneurysms with a headache of another cause. A strategy of primary CTA for diagnosis of SAH would be expected to subject many patients to unnecessary neurosurgical referrals for benign aneurysm, further procedures, and unnecessary contrast exposure. A CTA approach to diagnosing SAH may be appropriate in patients who refuse LP or have an unsuccessful LP.

- *Edlow JA, et al. Aneurysmal Subarachnoid Hemorrhage: Update for Emergency Physicians. J Emerg Med. 2008 Apr; 34(3): 237-51. full text*

#34

You are seeing a child that is 3 years old who is brought in by his parents for ataxia. His mental status is normal, he is afebrile, but there is some nystagmus and he has an unsteady, wide-based gait. According to the parents, he had a pruritic rash several days ago associated with URI symptoms, both of which self-resolved. The most likely diagnosis in this case is:

A. Drug ingestion

B. Neoplasm

C. Acute cerebellar ataxia

D. Acute postinfectious demyelinating encephalo-myelitis

E. Genetic ataxia syndrome (Friedreich's ataxia or ataxia telangiectasia)

#34

Answer: C

Acute cerebellar ataxia causes up to 40% of ataxic episodes in children. The disease is more common in males and more likely in the ages of 2-4 years old. Prior illness should heighten suspicion for the disease, and Varicella virus is the most common infectious cause. Current pathophysiology is thought to be due to autoimmune cerebellar demyelination.

On examination, patients will have truncal ataxia, and a wide based gait with a normal mental status. The differential should also include postinfectious demyelinating encephalitis, although mental status will be abnormal with encephalitis.

- *Rosen's Emergency Medicine - Concepts and Clinical Practice. 8th edition. 2013. Chapter 175: Neurologic Disorders. 2244-2245.*

#34

Current guidelines for the management of hypertension in patients with acute ischemic stroke recommend that antihypertensive treatment be reserved for those with markedly elevated blood pressures, unless fibrinolytic therapy is planned or indicated for treatment of another disease process. Which of the following would be one of these disease processes?

A. Angina

B. Diabetes out of control

C. Aortic dissection

D. Headache

E. Hypoxia with oxygen saturation less than 94% on room air

#34

Answer: C

The management of blood pressure in patients with acute ischemic stroke and CVA is controversial, although permissive hypertension is now widely accepted. Disease processes that would warrant immediate blood pressure control would include: aortic dissection, true hypertensive encephalopathy, and severe left ventricular heart failure.

- *Rosen's Emergency Medicine - Concepts and Clinical Practice. 8th edition. 2013. Chapter 101: Stroke. 1370-1371.*

#35

Several key features are necessary to make a diagnosis of delirium. Patients with delirium have disturbances in:

    A. Consciousness

    B. Cognition

    C. Perception

    D. All of the above

#35

Answer: D

Patients with delirium have disturbances in:

1. Consciousness
2. Cognition
3. Perception

Delirium develops over a short time course (hours to days) with initial manifestations being focus and attention. Patients can have mixed states of consciousness and waxing and waning symptoms. Cognitive deficiencies are generally disorientation and memory deficits. Perceptual disturbances include hallucinations or delusions.

- *Rosen's Emergency Medicine - Concepts and Clinical Practice. 8th edition. 2013. Chapter 104: Delirium and Dementia. 1398-1399.*

#36

Bilateral facial nerve paralysis as a presentation of Bell's palsy is rare but can occur with systemic infections. The two diseases that most commonly are associated with bilateral simultaneous onset of facial paralysis are:

A. Lyme disease and HIV

B. Syphilis and Lyme disease

C. HIV and Syphilis

D. Lyme disease and Infectious Mononucleosis

E. Infectious Mononucleosis and Syphilis

#36

Answer: D

Bilateral facial nerve paralysis is rare but can occur with systemic infections. The two diseases most commonly associated with bilateral simultaneous onset of facial paralysis are Lyme disease and infectious mononucleosis. Bilateral facial paralysis should be considered to be a manifestation of Lyme disease until further testing excludes this diagnosis.

- *Rosen's Emergency Medicine - Concepts and Clinical Practice. 8th edition. 2013. Chapter 105: Brain and Cranial Disorders. 1409-1417.*

#37

A radiologist calls you to inform you that a CT scan of the lumbar spine ordered by triage demonstrates findings consistent with "diskitis." True statements about diskitis include all of the following EXCEPT:

A. Treatment is primarily conservative with analgesics as an outpatient.

B. It is an infection of the nucleus pulposus, with secondary involvement of the cartilaginous endplate and vertebral body.

C. There is an increased incidence in immunocompromised patients.

D. Radicular symptoms are present in 50-90%, and the lumbar spine is the most common site of disease.

E. Fever is noted in more than 90%.

#37

Answer: A

With early IV antibiotics, outcomes are generally favorable, and S. aureus is the most common pathogen. Plain radiographs are often non-diagnostic. ESR can be elevated, raising further suspicion of disease. MRI is the diagnostic study of choice and can also exclude other diseases such as paravertebral or epidural abscess.

- *Rosen's Emergency Medicine - Concepts and Clinical Practice. 8th edition. 2013. Chapter 106: Spinal Cord Disorders. 1426.*

#38

With respect to the management of spontaneous ICH, which of the following statements is TRUE?

 A. Patients with ICH whose INR is elevated due to an warfarin should have their warfarin withheld, and must always receive prothrombin complex concentrates (PCC) instead of fresh frozen plasma (FFP).

 B. rFVIIa lowers the INR and if available, is recommended as a sole agent for OAC reversal in ICH.

 C. There is evidence that platelet transfusions in ICH patients with a history of antiplatelet use is beneficial.

 D. Patients with ICH should have intermittent pneumatic compression for prevention of venous thromboembolism.

 E. In patients with ICH, systolic blood pressure should not be lowered below 150/90 in order to preserve cerebral perfusion pressure.

#38

Answer: D

Patients with a severe coagulation factor deficiency or severe thrombocytopenia should receive appropriate factor replacement therapy or platelets. Patients with ICH whose INR is elevated due to warfarin should have their warfarin withheld, receive therapy to replace vitamin K-dependent factors (either PCC or FFP) and correct the INR, and receive intravenous vitamin K.

PCCs have NOT shown improved outcome compared with FFP. rFVIIa does not replace all factors and though INR may be lowered, clotting may not be restored in vivo; thus, rFVIIa is not routinely recommended as a sole agent for warfarin reversal. There is also an increase in thromboembolic risk with rFVIIa. The usefulness of platelet transfusions in ICH patients with a history of antiplatelet use is unclear and is considered investigational. In patients presenting with a systolic BP of 150 to 220mm Hg, acute lowering of systolic BP to 140 mm Hg is probably safe.

- *Morgenstern LB, et al. Guidelines for the management of spontaneous ICH: a guideline for healthcare professionals from the American Heart Association/American Stroke Association. Stroke. 2010 Sep;41(9): 2108-29. full text*

#39

With respect to the management of spontaneous ICH, which of the following statements is TRUE?

    A. Hyper or hypoglycemia has no detrimental effects on patients with ICH.

    B. Prophylactic anticonvulsant medications should always be given.

    C. Ventricular drainage as treatment for hydrocephalus is reasonable in patients with a depressed level of consciousness.

    D. New DNR discussions should occur immediately.

    E. None of the above

#39

Answer: C

Glucose should be monitored and normoglycemia is recommended. Although clinical seizures should be treated, the benefits of prophylactic anticonvulsant therapy remain unclear. Seizures may be harmful in patients with ICH, but anticonvulsants have not been demonstrated to statistically decrease the occurrence of seizure in ICH patients. Patients should be admitted to the intensive care unit after an ICH and discussions about DNR should be withheld until the second full day of hospitalization. After the acute period, a target of a target BP of <140/90 (<130/80 if diabetes or chronic kidney disease) is reasonable. Surgical interventions are appropriate in the patient with significant hydrocephalus and increasing risk or evidence of herniation.

• Morgenstern LB, et al. Guidelines for the management of spontaneous ICH: a guideline for healthcare professionals from the American Heart Association/American Stroke Association. Stroke. 2010 Sep;41(9): 2108-29. full text

#40

With respect to the management of spontaneous ICH, which of the following statements is TRUE? ICP monitoring should be considered in patients with:

A. GCS ≤ 8

B. Clinical evidence of transtentorial herniation

C. Significant intraventricular hemorrhage or hydrocephalus

D. All of the above

#40

Answer: D

Patients with a GCS ≤ 8, those with clinical evidence of transtentorial herniation, or those with significant IVH or hydrocephalus might be considered for ICP monitoring and treatment. A cerebral perfusion pressure of 50-70 mm Hg may be reasonable to maintain.

- *Morgenstern LB, et al. Guidelines for the management of spontaneous ICH: a guideline for healthcare professionals from the American Heart Association/American Stroke Association. Stroke. 2010 Sep;41(9): 2108-29. full text*

#41

You are seeing a 12 yo child with seizure disorders and a vagal nerve stimulator. What should you do if the patient and the parent senses that they are about to experience a seizure?

    A. Tap the subcutaneous device to activate it.

    B. Place a magnet over the device.

    C. Have the child drink some water.

    D. Administer an antiepileptic.

    E. None of the above

#41
Answer: B

Vagal nerve stimulators (VNS) are implantable devices used to prevent seizures and they are programmed to provide baseline intermittent stimulation of the left vagus nerve. Although the VNS delivers stimulation automatically in regular pulses all of the time, a magnet can be used to deliver extra electronic stimulation between cycles. The device can be activated by placing a hand held magnet over chest site. A magnet can also be used to stop the stimulation by persistently holding it over the device.

- *Rosen's Emergency Medicine - Concepts and Clinical Practice. 8th edition. 2013. Chapter 187: Evaluation of the Developmentally or Physically Disabled. 2409-2410.*

#42

Wernicke's encephalopathy is a clinical diagnosis. Which of the following is not part of the clinical features?

  A. Tremor

  B. Nutritional deficiency

  C. Ocular findings

  D. Ataxia

  E. Mental status changes

#42

Answer: A

Although many patients with Wernicke's encephalopathy may also be suffering from alcohol withdrawal, tremor is not part of the 4 general clinical features of the disease. The disease is caused by depletion of thiamine (Vitamin B1) stores.

Wernicke's should be considered in patients with 2 of the 4 clinical features of:

1. Nutritional deficiency
2. Ocular findings (bilateral 6th nerve or conjugate gaze palsy)
3. Ataxia
4. Mental status changes.

- *Rosen's Emergency Medicine - Concepts and Clinical Practice. 8th edition. 2013. Chapter 185: Alcohol Related Disease. 2381, 2386.*

#43

A patient has a seizure in the ED. He appeared postictal when you evaluate him, and you are asked by the nurse to see him one hour later, as he is complaining of short-ness of breath and is hypoxic to 87%. On examination, he has pulmonary rales in bilateral lung fields. What is the most likely cause of the hypoxia?

A. Neurogenic pulmonary edema

B. Bacterial pneumonia

C. Pulmonary embolism

D. Viral pneumonia

E. Exacerbation of his asthma

#43

Answer: A

Neurogenic pulmonary edema can occur after any CNS insult, including seizure, trauma, and hemorrhage. Although common, the disease progression does not usually cause severe respiratory distress. The excessive centrally mediated sympathetic discharge, vasoconstriction, and increased pulmonary capillary permeability can cause diffuse pulmonary edema. Most often, the neurogenic pulmonary edema that occurs post seizure is mistaken for aspiration pneumonia. Treatment should focus on increasing positive airway pressure, rather than on aggressive diuresis.

- *Rosen's Emergency Medicine - Concepts and Clinical Practice. 8th edition. 2013. Chapter 102: Seizure disorders. 1386-87.*

#44

Regarding cerebrospinal fluid analysis, which of the following is abnormal?

(Choose three answers.)

    A. The presence of > 1 polymononuclear neutrophil (PMN)

    B. Total white blood cell count of more than 5 cells/ mm^3

    C. The presence of an eosinophil

    D. The presence of a basophil

    E. All of the above

#44
Answer: A, B, and C

A healthy adult should not have any eosinophils in the CSF. The CSF is considered abnormal if there is more than

5 leukocytes/mm^3 with at most one granulocyte or PMN. Occasionally, basophils may be seen in the absence of disease.

- *Rosen's Emergency Medicine - Concepts and Clinical Practice. 8th edition. 2013. Chapter 109: Central Nervous System Infections. 1452-4.*

#45

Regarding concussion, which of the following statements is FALSE?

(Choose two answers.)

A. Concussion requires loss of consciousness (LOC).

B. Symptoms include headaches, fatigue, mood swings, neck pain, nausea and vomiting, dizziness, blurred vision, balance difficulty, photosensitivity, memory problems, difficulty concentrating, emotional lability, insomnia, depression and anxiety.

C. Most patients with concussion remain symptomatic for several months to years.

#45
Answer: A and C

Concussion can be graded by clinical manifestations and does not require LOC. There is often a transient LOC but it is not strictly required. Although most patients with concussion improve rapidly (within 3 weeks), a small percentage (approximately 10-20%) of those with sports-related concussion may remain symptomatic, particularly children and adolescents.

- *Zafonte R. Diagnosis and management of sports-related concussion. A 15 year old athlete with a concussion. JAMA. 2011 Jul 6; 306(1): 79-86. full text*

Amy Kaji

#46

Which of the following are TRUE about the management of concussion?

(Choose two answers.)

    A. A student with a concussion may return to play on the day of the injury if he passes a neurological test.

    B. The coach should evaluate players for concussion.

    C. A player with a potential concussion should be evaluated by a healthcare professional.

    D. Cervical spine injury should be excluded.

#46

Answer: C and D

According to the Zurich guidelines and the CDC, a player who shows any signs of a concussion should be evaluated by a healthcare professional on-site using a concussive injury tool such as SCAT3. Cervical spine injury should be excluded. If no healthcare provider is available, the player should receive urgent medical evaluation.

A player with a concussion should not return to play on the day of the injury. Coaches should not evaluate players for concussion. The coach's role is to remove the athlete from play, ensure that the athlete is evaluated by a healthcare professional, and to keep the athlete out of play until a health care professional states that the player is symptom free and may return to play.

.McCrory P, et al. Consensus statement on concussion in sport: the 4th International Conference on Concussion in Sport held in Zurich, November 2012. Br J Sports Med. 2013 Apr; 47(5): 250-8. full text

. CDC – Concussion http://www.cdc.gov/concussion/clinician.html

Amy Kaji

#47

Regarding the management of treatment after concussion, which of the following statements is TRUE?

(Choose three answers.)

   A. Physical rest is important.

   B. Rapid return to normal scholastic activities is encouraged.

   C. Adequate hydration may be helpful.

   D. Normalizing sleep patterns is important.

#47

Answer: A, C, and D

Symptomatic patients should be encouraged to rest rather than immediately return to any stressful activities. Neuropsychological testing may be necessary before full return to school. Additionally, medications that could result in rebound symptoms should also be avoided. In addition to sleep, proper nutrition, especially hydration, is important to improve recovery.

- *McCrory P, et al. Consensus statement on concussion in sport: the 4th International Conference on Concussion in Sport held in Zurich, November 2012. Br J Sports Med. 2013 Apr; 47(5): 250-8. full text*

- *CDC - Concussion http://www.cdc.gov/concussion/clinician.html*

#48

Regarding the treatment of migraine headaches in the emergency department (ED), which of the following is FALSE?

A. Patients may respond to metoclopramide or compazine in the ED.

B. Patients may respond to DHE 45 and metoclopramide.

C. Dexamethasone may be effective in reducing the risk of headache recurrence.

D. Ergotamine may be used to treat migraine headaches in the acute period.

E. It does not matter when treatment of the headache is initiated.

#48

Answer: E

For initial treatment of severe migraine, particularly if the migraine is accompanied by severe nausea or vomiting, intravenous metoclopramide or prochlorperazine may be effective. Parenteral DHE-45 should not be used as monotherapy; however oral DHE can be combined with metoclopramide. DHE-45 is contraindicated in patients with cardiac or cerebrovascular disease.

Adjunctive treatment with IV or intramuscular dexamethasone may reduce the risk of early headache recurrence. A single dose of dexamethasone may prevent short-term recurrence, resulting in less need for medication and fewer repeat visits to the office or emergency department. Abortive treatments, such as triptans, are usually more effective if given early in the course of the headache.

- *Rosen's Emergency Medicine - Concepts and Clinical Practice. 8th edition. 2013. Chapter 103: Headache Disorders. 1386-89.*

- *Singh A, et al. Does the addition of dexamethasone to standard therapy for acute migraine headache decrease the incidence of recurrent headache for patients treated in the emergency department? A meta-analysis and systematic review of the literature. Acad Emerg Med. 2008 Dec; 15(12): 1223-33. full text*

OBSTETRICS AND GYNECOLOGY

#1

Above what serum hCG level is the absence of intrauterine pregnancy by transvaginal ultrasound (and no fluid in the pouch of Douglass or an ectopic mass) presumptive evidence of ectopic pregnancy?

A. 300

B. 400

C. 1000

D. 2000

E. 600

#1

Answer: D

Mol, et al found that a hCG above 1,500 mIU/mL in the presence of sonographic abnormalities such as fluid in the pouch of Douglas or an ectopic mass was presumptive diagnosis of an ectopic pregnancy. For patients **without these sonographic abnormalities, a serum hCG level greater than 2,000 mIU/mL increased the likelihood of ectopic pregnancy.**

Close outpatient follow-up for repeat examination and ultrasound is necessary in all in hemodynamically stable patients without active bleeding with no increasing pain, who have non-diagnostic ultrasounds and hCG levels greater than 2,000 mIU/mL.

- *LLSA 2007: Clinical policy: Critical issues in the initial evaluation and management of patients presenting to the emergency department in early pregnancy. Ann Emerg Med. 2003 Jan; 41(1): 123-33. full text*

#2

What is the frequency of treatment success in methotrexate therapy for ectopic pregnancy in carefully selected patients?

    A. 1-3%

    B. 30-40%

    C. 55-64%

    D. 64-94%

    E. 96-99%

Amy Kaji

#2

Answer: D

Selected patients with close follow-up have been safely treated with methotrexate, with **success rates ranging from 64% to 94%.** A study of 120 women diagnosed with ectopic pregnancy were treated as outpatients with methotrexate with successes correlated with the following criteria:

- An unruptured ectopic mass less than 3.5 cm in size
- Hemodynamic stability
- Absence of active bleeding or signs of hemoperitoneum.

In 1996, Stitka, et al reviewed the cases of 50 women with ectopic pregnancy treated with methotrexate administered intramuscularly. The success rate was 65% with the first injection and 78% with a second injection.

In 1998 and 1999, Lipscomb, et al. reviewed the cases of over 300 women with ectopic pregnancy treated with methotrexate showing overall success rates without surgical intervention of 90.1% - 91%. The factor most associated with failure after 1 dose of methotrexate was an elevated hCG level greater than 10,000 mIU/mL.

Stitka, et al and Lipscomb, et al demonstrated increased success rates if no fetal cardiac activity was detected. Although methotrexate is a feasible outpatient treatment strategy, ED prescription and arrangement of follow-up is often outside the abilities of the ED physician. Thus, it should only be performed in the setting of an OBGYN consult in hemodynamically stable patients with the above criteria.

- *Lipscomb GH, et al. Analysis of three hundred fifteen ectopic pregnancies treated with single-dose methotrexate. Am J Obstet Gynecol. 1998 Jun; 178(6): 1354-8.*

- *Stitka CS, et al. Single dose methotrexate for the treatment of ectopic pregnancy: Northwestern Memorial Hospital three-year experience. Am J Obstet Gynecol. 1996 Jun; 174(6): 1840-6.*

#3

Most breast abscesses occur 1 to 3 months postpartum, but post-menopausal women may also develop mastitis and abscesses. Which of the following are common to both types?

A. The abscesses are often found in the subareolar region in association with duct ectasia.

B. Causative bacteria are most commonly E coli and group D strep.

C. Staph species are found in both abscess types.

D. Klebsiella is a causative species.

E. Infection is most often located away from the areola.

#3

Answer: C

Staph species are found in both postpartum and post-menopausal breast abscesses. Postpartum abscesses are caused by normal skin pathogens that invade through cracks in the nipple, and breast milk is an ideal culture medium. Unrecognized infection then forms an abscess, usually located away from the areola. Staph are the most common causative agents. Preventive measures include nipple hygiene, hand washing, cleansing of the infant's skin and early recognition.

Postmenopausal abscesses differ in cause and presentation. Causative bacteria include E coli, Group D Strep, Staph, and anaerobes. These abscesses are most often found in the sub-areolar region due to chronic inflammation of ducts. Recurrence rates after simple incision and drainage can be as great as 40%.

- *Eryilmaz R, Sahin M, Hakan Tekelioglu M, Daldal E. Management of lactational breast abscesses. Breast. Oct 2005;14(5):375-9.*

- *Dixon JM. Outpatient treatment of non-lactational breast abscesses. Br J Surg. Jan 1992;79(1):56-7.*

#4

You are practicing in a rural ED without immediate obstetric back-up. A patient presents with a delivering fetus with shoulder dystocia. All of the following maneuvers may be helpful EXCEPT:

A. Hyperextend the mother's legs

B. Deliver the posterior shoulder first

C. Perform an episiotomy

D. Have an assistant apply suprapubic pressure in an attempt to dislodge the impacted fetal shoulder.

E. Place the laboring mother on her hands and knees (the all-fours maneuver).

#4

Answer: A

Hyperflexion of the maternal thighs onto the abdomen may be attempted, but hyperextension has not been demonstrated to be helpful. The all-fours maneuver resulted in an 83% success rate in one series. Disagreement exists about which maneuver, or series of maneuvers is likely to be the most successful. However, it is important to be able to perform multiple techniques in the setting of a complicated delivery.

- *Roberts and Hedges' Clinical Procedures in Emergency Medicine. 6th edition. 2013. Chapter 56: Emergency Childbirth. 1155-1179.*

#5

Metrorrhagia is bleeding at irregular intervals other than the usual time of menstruation, and may represent an anovulatory disorder. All of the following are causes of anovulatory bleeding EXCEPT:

A. Polycystic ovarian syndrome

B. Poorly controlled diabetes

C. Von Willebrand's disease (VWD)

D. Primary ovarian dysfunction

E. Hyperprolactinemia

#5

Answer: C

VWD represents a disorder of hemostasis. Other etiologies of anovulatory bleeding include hypothyroidism, Cushing's, Addison's and Congenital Adrenal Hyperplasia.

- *Bayer SR, DeCherney AH. Clinical manifestations and treatment of dysfunctional uterine bleeding. JAMA. Apr 14 1993;269(14):1823-8.*

#6

Ectopic pregnancy results from implantation of a fertilized ovum at a site other than the endometrium of the uterus. The most frequent site of implantation is:

    A. The lateral two-thirds of the fallopian tube

    B. The medial one-third of the fallopian tube

    C. Interstitial or corneal

    D. Within the ovary

    E. In the abdomen

#6

Answer: A

The most frequent site of implantation is the lateral 2/3 of the fallopian tube (80%). 15% of ectopic pregnancies implant in the medial 1/3 of the fallopian tube; interstitial or cornual implantation occurs in approximately 3%; and interstitial and cornual implantations carry the greatest risk of mortality because of their hemorrhagic tendencies. Extratubal pregnancies occur in 5%: within the abdomen in 2%, and in the ovary in 3%.

- *Farquhar CM. Ectopic pregnancy. Lancet. 2005 Aug 13-19; 366(9485): 583-91.*

#7

There are multiple risk factors for ectopic pregnancy, such as one or more episodes of salpingitis, the use of an IUD associated with a pregnancy (14% of women who become pregnant with an IUD have an ectopic), prior tubal sterilization associated with a pregnancy (16% of women who become pregnant after being sterilized have an ectopic), and a history of a prior ectopic pregnancy. Approximately what proportion of women diagnosed with an ectopic pregnancy DO NOT have risk factors?

    A. 5%

    B. 10%

    C. 20%

    D. 40%

    E. 60%

#7

Answer: D

Up to 42% of women with ectopic pregnancy have no historic risk factors. Ectopic pregnancy after tubal sterilization is thought to represent partial recanalization with access of the sperm to the ovum but impaired passage of the fertilized ovum to the uterine cavity. Similar to patients with intrauterine devices, patients who have had prior tubal sterilization have a delay in diagnosis.

- *Mol BW, van Der Veen F, Bossuyt PM. Implementation of probabilistic decision rules improves the predictive values of algorithms in the diagnostic management of ectopic pregnancy. Hum Reprod. 1999 Nov; 14(11): 2855-62. full text*

Amy Kaji

#8

Empiric treatment of PID is recommended in women at risk for STDs with pelvic pain, if no cause for the illness other than PID can be identified. Which of the following criteria should be met?

A. Cervical motion tenderness

B. Uterine tenderness

C. Adnexal tenderness

D. If any one of the above are present

#8

Answer: D

Empiric treatment of PID should be initiated in sexually active young women and other women at risk for STDs if they are experiencing pelvic or lower abdominal pain, if no cause for the illness other than PID can be identified, and if ONE or more of the following minimum criteria are present on pelvic examination:

1. Cervical motion tenderness

2. Uterine tenderness

3. Adnexal tenderness.

The requirement that all three minimum criteria be present before the initiation of empiric treatment could result in insufficient sensitivity for the diagnosis of PID. The presence of signs of lower genital tract inflammation, in addition to one of the three minimum criteria, increases the specificity of diagnosis.

The following additional criteria can be used to enhance the specificity of the minimum criteria and support a diagnosis of PID although most ED physicians will opt to base treatment on clinical grounds:

1. Oral temperature >101°F (>38.3°C)

2. Abnormal cervical or vaginal mucopurulent discharge,

3. Presence of abundant numbers of WBC on saline microscopy of vaginal secretions,

4. Elevated erythrocyte sedimentation rate,

5. Elevated C-reactive protein, and

6. Laboratory documentation of cervical infection with N. gonorrhoeae or C. trachomatis.

Amy Kaji

- *CDC - PID Guidelines http://www.cdc.gov/std/treatment/2010/pid.htm*

#9

There has been a persistent trend toward outpatient treatment of PID with only 10 to 25% of women now being hospitalized. The CDC recommends that the decision to hospitalize for PID should be individualized and at the discretion of the clinician. The CDC's recommended indications for hospitalization include all of the following EXCEPT:

A. Pregnancy

B. Tubo-ovarian abscess

C. Lack of response to oral medications

D. Severe clinical illness

E. HIV positivity

#9

Answer: E

Recommended indications for hospitalization include:

1. Pregnancy
2. Lack of response or tolerance to oral medications
3. Nonadherence to therapy
4. Inability to take oral medications due to nausea and vomiting
5. Severe clinical illness (high fever, nausea, vomiting, severe abdominal pain)
6. Pelvic abscess, including tuboovarian abscess
7. Possible need for surgical intervention or diagnostic exploration for alternative etiology (eg, appendicitis)

There are also no data suggesting that HIV-infected women have a worse or different clinical response to PID therapy.

- *CDC PID http://www.cdc.gov/std/treatment/2010/pid.htm*

- *Walker, CK, Wiesenfeld, HC. Antibiotic therapy for acute pelvic inflammatory disease: the 2006 Centers for Disease Control and Prevention sexually transmitted diseases treatment guidelines. Clin Infect Dis 2007; 44 Suppl 3:S111 full text*

#10

Regarding ovarian torsion, which of the following statements is FALSE?

A. Ovarian torsion may occur in all ages.

B. Ovarian torsion may occur in a normal ovary.

C. The gold standard for diagnosis is ultrasound

D. The clinical diagnosis of ovarian torsion should be considered in women with the lower abdominal or pelvic pain and an ovarian cyst or mass.

E. Expedient diagnosis of ovarian torsion is important to preserve ovarian function and prevent necrosis, infarction, or systemic infection.

Amy Kaji

#10

Answer: C

Ovarian torsion occurs in all age groups and may occur in a normal ovary. The gold standard for diagnosis is surgery. Three-dimensional (3D) ultrasound or two-dimensional ultrasound with Doppler is useful for preoperative imaging of the adnexa when torsion is suspected. However, torsion can be intermittent and may not be detected on a pelvic ultrasound. A definitive diagnosis of ovarian torsion is based upon surgical findings.

- *Rosen's Emergency Medicine - Concepts and Clinical Practice. 8th edition. 2013. Chapter 100: Selected Gynecologic Disorders. 1355-1358.*

#11

Which of the following types of deliveries predisposes to the highest risk of postpartum endometritis?

A. Elective caesarean delivery

B. Emergency caesarean delivery

C. Emergency vaginal delivery

D. Induced vaginal delivery

E. Natural vaginal delivery

#11

Answer: B

Cesarean delivery is the most important risk factor for development of postpartum endometritis. The rates of endometritis (in the absence of antibiotic prophylaxis) after non elective cesarean, elective cesarean, and vaginal delivery are about 30%, 7%, and less than 3% respectively. Additional risk factors for postpartum endometritis include:

1. Prolonged labor
2. Prolonged rupture of membranes
3. Multiple cervical examinations
4. Internal fetal or uterine monitoring
5. Large amount of meconium in amniotic fluid
6. Manual removal of the placenta
7. Low socioeconomic status
8. Maternal diabetes mellitus or severe anemia
9. Preterm birth
10. Bacterial vaginosis
11. Operative vaginal delivery
12. Postterm pregnancy
13. HIV infection
14. Colonization with group B streptococcus

- *Rosen's Emergency Medicine - Concepts and Clinical Practice. 8th edition. 2013. Chapter 181: Labor and Delivery And Their Complications. 2350.*

#12

You are called to the parking lot for a woman who is delivering her baby in the car. You are able to assist her into the ED and safely deliver the baby. Within a few minutes after the placenta is removed, the mother begins to hemorrhage, and you believe that she has a uterine inversion. There is no obstetrician in the house. You should do all of the following EXCEPT:

A. Attempt manual replacement of the uterus.

B. Administer uterotonic agents, such as oxytocin.

C. Administer two large bore IVs and begin administering blood.

D. After hemodynamic stabilization is achieved, administer intravenous nitroglycerine.

E. After hemodynamic stabilization is achieved, administer terbutaline.

#12

Answer: B

Interventions for the management of acute uterine inversion should begin promptly and simultaneously. Uterotonic drugs should be discontinued since uterine relaxation is needed for replacement of uterus. Intravenous access and aggressive fluid resuscitation is critical. An immediate attempt to manually replace the inverted uterus to its normal position should be made. This is best accomplished by placing a hand inside the vagina and pushing the fundus cephalad along the long axis of the vagina. Prompt intervention is important since the lower uterine segment and cervix contract over time, thus making manual replacement progressively more difficult.

When immediate uterine replacement is unsuccessful, pharmacologic agents should be given to relax the uterus. Manual replacement should then reattempted. Possible pharmacological options for relaxation are:

- Nitroglycerine: 50 to 500 micrograms are intravenously, followed by up to three additional doses of 50 to 250 micrograms, as needed. (Caution should be given in actively bleeding and hemodynamically unstable patients.)

- Terbutaline 0.25 milligrams intravenously or subcutaneously

- Magnesium 4 to 6 grams intravenously over 15 to 20 minutes

Both terbutaline and magnesium have relatively mild effects on the myometrium and magnesium sulfate has a slow onset of action.

- *Rosen's Emergency Medicine - Concepts and Clinical Practice. 8th edition. 2013. Chapter 181: Labor and Delivery And Their Complications. 2349.*

#13

Regarding pelvic inflammatory disease (PID), which of the following is NOT a criteria for which hospitalization should be considered?

A. Pregnancy

B. Tuboovarian abscess

C. Vaginal bleeding

D. A surgical emergency can not be excluded (e.g., appendicitis).

E. The patient is unable to tolerate an outpatient oral regimen.

#13

Answer: C

Criteria for which hospitalization includes:

1. Pregnancy
2. Surgical emergency can't be excluded
3. Failure of oral antimicrobial therapy
4. Unable to follow or tolerate an outpatient regimen
5. Severe illness, nausea and vomiting, or high fever
6. Tuboovarian abscess

• *CDC - Pelvic Inflammatory Disease http://www.cdc.gov/std/treatment/2010/pid.htm*

#14

A 30 year old G4P4 patient who is postpartum day #3 presents with subjective fevers, abdominal pain, and foul smelling lochia. You suspect postpartum endometritis. All of the following are risk factors for endometritis, EXCEPT:

A. Operative delivery

B. Prolonged rupture of membranes

C. Prolonged stage 2 of labor

D. Frequent or excessive pelvic examinations

E. Urinary tract infection in the third trimester

#14

Answer: E

All of the above, except urinary tract infections are associated with postpartum endometritis. Causative organisms for these infections include gram-negative coliforms, bacteroides, and streptococci. Infection occurs when these bacteria invade the uterus or other tissues along the birth canal. Classic features, such as foul odor discharge, fever and abdominal pain develop on the second or third day postpartum. A search for retained products of conception is required, especially if bleeding is ongoing. Most patients require admission and treatment with clindamycin and an aminoglycoside, or second or third generation cephalosporin.

- *Rosen's Emergency Medicine - Concepts and Clinical Practice. 8th edition. 2013. Chapter 181: Labor and Delivery And Their Complications. 2350.*

#15

About 0.4 to 1.3% of pregnant women have asthma. Which of the following statements is FALSE about asthma during pregnancy?

A. Asthma improves during pregnancy in over 90% of patients.

B. Asthma therapy during pregnancy is directed at providing adequate oxygenation for both mother and fetus.

C. The management of pregnant asthmatics is essentially the same as that for non-pregnant asthmatics.

D. Inhaled beta agonists and corticosteroids appear to be safe in pregnancy.

E. Theophylline is category C in pregnancy.

#15

Answer: A

- One third of pregnant patients with asthma improve during pregnancy, one third remain unchanged, and one third become worse. The other statements are true. Theophylline is a pregnancy category C medication. The following are pregnancy risk categories for medications.

- Category A - Adequate and well-controlled studies have failed to demonstrate a risk to the fetus in the first trimester of pregnancy (and there is no evidence of risk in later trimesters).

- Category B - Animal studies have failed to demonstrate a risk to the fetus and there are no adequate and well-controlled studies in pregnant women.

- Category C - Animal studies have shown an adverse effect on the fetus and there are no adequate and well-controlled studies in humans, but potential benefits may warrant use of the drug in pregnant women despite potential risks.

- Category D - There is positive evidence of human fetal risk based on adverse reaction data from investigational or marketing experience or studies in humans, but potential benefits may warrant use of the drug in pregnant women despite potential risks.

- Category X -Studies in animals or humans have demonstrated fetal abnormalities and/or there is positive evidence of human fetal risk based on adverse reaction data from investigational or marketing experience, and the risks involved in use of the drug in pregnant women clearly outweigh potential benefits.

- Category N - FDA has not classified the drug.

. *Rey E, Boulet LP. Asthma in pregnancy. BMJ. Mar 17 2007; 334(7593):582-5*

#16

A 22 year old female present with vaginal bleeding and pelvic pain. She thinks she is 7 weeks pregnant by LMP. She has not had an ultrasound confirming an intrauterine pregnancy. You express your concern for an ectopic pregnancy. What would NOT be accurate to tell her about ectopic pregnancies?

A. Ectopic pregnancies are the third leading cause of maternal death.

B. Intrauterine devices (IUDs and previous ectopic pregnancies are risk factors for ectopic pregnancies.

C. The risk of having an ectopic pregnancy after a prior ectopic is 22%.

D. Predisposing risk factors for ectopic pregnancy are present in nearly all ectopic pregnancies.

E. Tubal surgeries and assisted reproductive technology are risk factors for ectopic pregnancies.

#16

Answer: D

Risk factors for ectopic pregnancy are absent in almost half of patients. Risk factors for ectopic pregnancy include tubal surgery, PID, smoking, advanced age, prior spontaneous abortion, medically induced abortion, history of infertility, and IUD. Adnexal masses are palpated only 10-20% of the time. Ectopic pregnancies occur in approximately 1% of all pregnancies with 98% of those implanting in the fallopian tubes. Prior ectopic pregnancy increases the risk for recurrence, and PID increases a person's risk 7-fold.

- *Rosen's Emergency Medicine - Concepts and Clinical Practice. 8th edition. 2013. Chapter 33: Acute Pelvic Pain in Women. 2350.*

#17

You are in the ER when suddenly a man bursts in and says he thinks his wife about to deliver a baby in the car. You run out to the parking lot to find a woman in the backseat with the fetal head at the perineum. As you begin to attempt to deliver the fetus with slight traction on the head, you realize neither shoulder is able to be delivered. Which of the following are included in your approach to dealing with shoulder dystocia:

A. Call for backup (obstetrics/neonatology)

B. Episiotomy

C. Flex mother's legs and apply suprapubic pressure

D. Corkscrew the shoulders

E. All the above

#17

Answer: E

Management using the HELPER mnemonic successfully delivers almost all cases of shoulder dystocia.

H - call for **help**

E - **episiotomy** (or episioproctotomy) to increase the anteroposterior diameter of passage

L - **legs** flexed (McRoberts maneuver)

P - **pressure** applied suprapubically and Rubin's maneuver (applying shoulder pressure to the fetus to decreases the biacromial diameter)

E - **enter** the vagina and attempt Wood's corkscrew maneuver by pushing the most accessible shoulder toward the chest to corkscrew the shoulders through the canal

R - **remove** posterior arm by sweeping it across the chest and bring fetal hand to the chin, grasp and pull out of the birth canal and across the face.

• Rosen's Emergency Medicine - Concepts and Clinical Practice. 8th edition. 2013. Chapter 181: Labor and Delivery and Their Complications. 2345.

#18

Which of the following is NOT an ABSOLUTE or RELA-TIVE contraindication for use of methotrexate (MTX) for the medical treatment of ectopic pregnancy?

A. Hemodynamic instability

B. hCG of 2000 mIU/mL

C. Ectopic mass of 6cm

D. 300 ml of free fluid in the pelvis

E. Cardiac activity

#18

Answer: B

MTX treatment of ectopic pregnancy should be reserved for patients with high compliance, close followup, hemodynamically stable, with a hCG concentration ≤5000 mIU/mL, and no fetal cardiac activity.

High hCG levels and fetal cardiac activity have been shown in studies to predict the need for multiple doses and treatment failure. Ectopic mass size less than 3 to 4 cm is also commonly used as a patient selection criterion; however, this has not been confirmed as a predictor of successful treatment. It should be noted that MTX is renally cleared, and in women with renal insufficiency, a single dose of MTX can lead to death or severe complications, including bone marrow suppression, ARDS and bowel ischemia.

Some women are not appropriate candidates for medical therapy and should be managed surgically, including women with the following characteristics:

1. Hemodynamically unstable
2. Signs of impending or ongoing ectopic mass rupture (ie, severe or persistent abdominal pain or >300 mL of free peritoneal fluid outside the pelvic cavity)
3. Clinically important abnormalities in hematologic, renal or hepatic lab values
4. Immunodeficiency
5. Active pulmonary disease
6. Peptic ulcer disease
7. Hypersensitivity to MTX
8. Coexistent viable intrauterine pregnancy
9. Breastfeeding

10. Unwilling or unable to be compliant with post-therapeutic monitoring

11. Do not have timely access to a medical institution.

• *Menon S, et al. Establishing a human chorionic gonadotropin cutoff to guide methotrexate treatment of ectopic pregnancy: A systematic review. Fertil Steril. 2007 Mar; 87(3): 481-4.*

• *Bachman E, Barnhart K. Medical Management of Ectopic Pregnancy: A Comparison of Regimens. Clin Obstet Gynecol. 2012; 55(2): 440–447.*

#19

You are seeing a 50 year old female with a complaint of profuse vaginal bleeding. You suspect abnormal uterine bleeding (AUB). True statements about AUB include all of the following EXCEPT:

A. Approximately 10% of AUB results from anovulation, and 90% occur with ovulatory cycles.

B. In ovulatory AUB, irregular shedding of the endometrium is related to a constant low level of estrogen that causes endometrial growth that then degenerates and results in spotting.

C. Obese females tend to have irregularities in their menstrual cycles due to non-ovarian endogenous production of estrogen often related to their degree of adipose tissue. This usually results in prolonged cycles of amenorrhea that alternate with cycles of metrorrhagia or menometrorrhagia.

D. Although AUB in itself is rarely fatal, outpatient workup will focus on identifying a cause and differentiating it from endometrial cancer, particularly in postmenopausal women.

E. AUB is most common at the extreme ages of a woman's reproductive years.

#19

Answer: A

Approximately 90% of DUB results from anovulation, and 10% occur with ovulatory cycles. During an anovulatory cycle, the corpus luteum fails to form, causing failure of normal progesterone secretion. The result is unopposed estradiol production and increasing growth of the endometrium. Without progesterone, the endometrium proliferates and eventually outgrows its blood supply, leading to necrosis. The end result is overproduction of uterine blood flow. Most severe cases of AUB occur in adolescent girls during the first 18 months after the onset of menstruation, when their immature hypothalamic-pituitary axis may fail to respond to estrogen and progesterone, resulting in anovulation.

- *Bayer SR, DeCherney AH. Clinical manifestations and treatment of dysfunctional uterine bleeding. JAMA. Apr 14 1993; 269(14): 1823-8.*

#20

You are seeing a 27 year old female in whom you suspect ovarian torsion. True statements about this entity include all of the following EXCEPT:

A. Classically, patients present with sudden onset, severe, unilateral lower abdominal pain that worsens intermittently over many hours.

B. Fever may occur as a late finding as the ovary becomes necrotic.

C. A unilateral, tender adnexal mass has been reported in between 50 and 90% of patients. However, absence of such a finding does not exclude the diagnosis.

D. Torsion of a normal ovary does not occur.

E. Computed tomography may demonstrate an enlarged ovary and adnexal masses but is unable to evaluate the presence or absence of blood flow to the involved ovary.

#20
Answer: D

Multiple factors have been found to be responsible for the development of ovarian torsion. Torsion is rare in a normal ovary and more frequently arises from one of many anatomic changes. Torsion of a normal ovary is most common among young children, in whom developmental abnormalities such as excessively long fallopian tubes or absent mesosalpinx may be responsible. In fact, less than half of torsed ovaries in pediatric patients involve cysts, teratomas, or other masses. During early pregnancy, the presence of an enlarged corpus luteum cyst predisposes the ovary to torsion. Women undergoing induction of ovulation for infertility carry an even greater risk, as numerous theca lutein cysts significantly expand the ovarian volume.

Ovarian tumors and cysts, both benign and malignant, are implicated in 50-60% of cases of torsion. Involved masses are nearly all greater than 4-6 cm, although torsion is possible with smaller masses. CT may be useful in ruling out other possible causes of lower abdominal pain in cases of diagnostic uncertainty. Additionally, CT can exclude the presence of a pelvic mass, which greatly adds in the ability to rule out torsion.

- *Rosen's Emergency Medicine - Concepts and Clinical Practice. 8th edition. 2013. Chapter 100: Selected Gynecologic Disorders. 1355-1358.*

#21

Regarding Pelvic Inflammatory Disease (PID), which of the following statements is FALSE?

A. Up to 1 % of women with untreated gonorrhea and 20% of women with untreated chlamydia infection may develop PID.

B. Quinolones, such as levofloxacin and ciprofloxacin are first-line agents in treating gonorrhea.

C. The spectrum of antibiotic coverage must include Chlamydia trachomatis and Neisseria gonorrhoeae, Streptococci, gram-negative enteric bacilli, and anaerobes.

D. The optimal duration of therapy is unknown, although the CDC recommend 14 days of doxycycline treatment.

E. Male sex partners of women with PID should be examined and treated if they had sexual contact with the patient during the previous 60 days prior to the patient's onset of symptoms.

#21

Answer: B

Due to the rising levels of fluoroquinolone resistance among Neisseria gonorrhoeae isolates, the CDC no longer recommends the use of fluoroquinolones for the treatment of gonorrhea infections, including associated conditions, such as PID.

Recommended regimens include:

- Ceftriaxone (250 mg intramuscularly in a single dose) plus doxycycline (100 mg orally twice a day for 14 days) with or without metronidazole (500 mg orally twice a day for 14 days).

- Cefoxitin (2 g intramuscularly in a single dose) concurrently with probenecid (1 g orally in a single dose) plus doxycycline (100 mg orally twice a day for 14 days) with or without metronidazole (500 mg orally twice a day for 14 days).

- Other parenteral third-generation cephalosporins, such as cefotaxime (1 gram intramuscularly in a single dose) or ceftizoxime (1 gram intramuscularly in a single dose) plus doxycycline (100 mg orally twice a day for 14 days) with or without metronidazole (500 mg orally twice a day for 14 days).

The decision to add metronidazole is based upon clinical assessment of the risk of anaerobic organisms in the individual patient. For example, the addition of metronidazole may be considered in patients with:

- Pelvic abscess

- Proven or suspected infection with Trichomonas vaginalis or bacterial vaginosis

- History of gynecological instrumentation in the

preceding two to three weeks

- *CDC - PID Guidelines http://www.cdc.gov/std/treatment/2010/pid.htm*

#22

You are seeing a 29 year old female who is postpartum day 8. She presents with fever, uterine tenderness, foul lochia, and some mild vaginal bleeding. You suspect postpartum endometritis. What is the most important risk factor for this entity?

    A. History of Group B strep colonization

    B. History of pelvic inflammatory disease

    C. History of preterm labor

    D. History of cesarean section

    E. History of bacterial vaginosis

#22

Answer: D

Cesarean delivery is the most important risk factor for development of postpartum endometritis. The rates of endometritis after nonelective cesarean are higher than those in, elective cesarean or vaginal delivery

Additional risk factors for postpartum endometritis include:

- Prolonged labor

- Prolonged rupture of membranes

- Multiple cervical examinations

- Internal fetal or uterine monitoring

- Large amount of meconium in amniotic fluid

- Manual removal of the placenta

- Low socioeconomic status

- Maternal diabetes mellitus or severe anemia

- Preterm birth

- Bacterial vaginosis

- Operative vaginal delivery

- Postterm pregnancy

- HIV infection

- Colonization with group B streptococcus.

. Watts D. et al. Bacterial vaginosis as a risk factor for post-cesarean endometritis. Obstet Gynecol. 1990 Jan; 75(1): 52-8.

. Smaill F. Hofmeyr GJ. Antibiotic prophylaxis for cesarean section. Cochrane Database Syst Rev. 2002;(3):CD000933.

#23

You are seeing a 34 year old G5P4 obese female and (with history of asthma) who is 38 weeks by dates, and she complains of shortness of breath and dry cough. Which of the following should be part of your differential diagnosis?

A. Asthma exacerbation

B. Decreased functional residual capacity due to gravid uterus and obesity

C. Pulmonary embolus

D. Peripartum cardiomyopathy (PPCM)

E. Viral URI

F. All of the above

#23

Answer: F

Four criteria are needed to meet the definition of peripartum cardiomyopathy:

1. Development of cardiac failure in the last month of pregnancy or within five months of delivery

2. Absence of an identifiable cause for the cardiac failure

3. Absence of recognizable heart disease prior to the last month of pregnancy

4. LV systolic dysfunction (eg, left ventricular ejection fraction [LVEF] below 45%)

Women who develop cardiomyopathy earlier in pregnancy do not meet the definition of PPCM based upon the first and third criteria; however, the disease process is probably the same. The characteristics of early-onset disease were evaluated in a review of 123 women with a history of cardiomyopathy diagnosed during pregnancy. One hundred women met the traditional criteria for PPCM, presenting at a mean of 38 weeks, and 23 presented earlier at a mean of 32 weeks. There were no differences between the two groups in terms of age, race, associated conditions, LVEF (29 versus 27%), the rate and time of recovery, and maternal outcomes. These observations suggest that patients with an early presentation may be part of the spectrum of PPCM. However, always consider other causes of shortness of breath in pregnant and postpartum patients, such as pulmonary embolism.

- *Elkayam U. et al. Pregnancy-associated cardiomyopathy: clinical characteristics and a comparison between early and late presentation. Circulation. 2005 Apr 26; 111(16): 2050-5. full text*

#24

Your patient with an ectopic pregnancy wants to know if she is a candidate for non-surgical treatment. Which of the following statements about methotrexate for ectopic pregnancy is TRUE?

(Choose two answers.)

- A. All ectopic pregnancies should be treated initially with methotrexate.

- B. To be eligible, the non-ruptured ectopic pregnancy should be no greater than 1 cm.

- C. To be eligible, the hCG should be < 1000 IU/L.

- D. The presence of fetal cardiac activity is a relative contraindication.

- E. To be eligible, the patient must be hemodynamically stable, be reliable, and be amenable to the treatment regimen.

#24

Answer: D and E

The hCG should be < 5000 IU/L. The overall success rate for methotrexate is 89%. Patients may experience transient abdominal pain within 3-7 days after the start of treatment classified as separation pain. If the pain progresses in severity, is persistent, or is accompanied by other signs and symptoms, treatment failure or rupture of the ectopic should be suspected. The most common side effects from methotrexate are stomatitis, nausea, vomiting, and dizziness. If the patient meets criteria for methotrexate, baseline liver function tests should be ordered. The single-dose regimen involves methotrexate 50 mg IM on day 1 and on day 7 if the hCG decreases by less than 15% between days 4 and 7. The presence of fetal cardiac activity is a relative contraindication, as it is associated with high failure rates. An ectopic size > 3 cm is also associated with higher methotrexate failure rates.

- Menon S, et al. Establishing a human chorionic gonadotropin cutoff to guide methotrexate treatment of ectopic pregnancy: A systematic review. Fertil Steril. 2007 Mar; 87(3): 481-4.

- Bachman E, Barnhart K. Medical Management of Ectopic Pregnancy: A Comparison of Regimens. Clin Obstet Gynecol. 2012; 55(2): 440–447. full text

#25

You are seeing a G1P0 patient who is 10 3/7 weeks pregnant with vaginal bleeding. She has not previously had an ultrasound confirming an intrauterine pregnancy. Which of the following sites would be more likely to be misdiagnosed as intrauterine?

A. Fallopian tube

B. Fimbriae

C. Ovary

D. Interstitial

#25

Answer: D

An interstitial pregnancy implants in the myometrium in the proximal portion of the fallopian tube. Although 0.7mm wide and 1-2 cm long, this area is more distensible than the fallopian tube and typically presents after 8 weeks' gestation. Due to the eccentricity of the interstitial pregnancy and implantation in the uterine myometrium it can easily be misdiagnosed on ultrasound for an intrauterine pregnancy.

Criteria that can aid in the differentiation of an interstitial ectopic from intrauterine pregnancy include:

1. An empty uterus
2. Gestational sac seen separate from the endometrium
3. Gestational sac > 1cm away from the lateral edge of the uterine cavity
4. <5 mm mantle surrounding the sac

Rupture may occur as early as 5 weeks gestation. Maternal mortality rate for interstitial ectopic pregnancy is 2-3%. Interstitial ectopic pregnancy is diagnosed on ultrasound in only 65% of cases, and laparoscopy remains the most accurate tool.

The most common location for ectopic pregnancy is the fallopian tube. The least common location is the cervical region, but is as high as 9.8% after assisted reproductive treatment, specifically IVF. Although very rare, diagnosis of cervical ectopic pregnancy is also often delayed due to decreased accuracy of ultrasound.

• *Williams Obstetrics 24th edition. 2014. Chapter 19: Ectopic Pregnancy. 377-392.*

#26
Which of the following is NOT a known risk factor for ectopic pregnancy?

A. Prior ectopic pregnancy

B. Prior sexually transmitted disease

C. Tubal infection or pelvic adhesions

D. Assisted reproductive treatment (ART)

E. Increased maternal age

F. All of the above

#26

Answer: F

All of these listed are known risk factors. However, 40-50% of patients with confirmed ectopic pregnancy have no risk factors, so the absence of such factors does not rule out the diagnosis. The incidence is as high as 20% in patients who have had a prior tubal surgery, and ART is a well-established risk factor. According to the CDC, women 35-44 had the highest rates of ectopic pregnancy when compared to patients in the 15-24 year old groups, possibly because these older patients may be exposed to more risk factors with increasing age.

- *Farquhar CM. Ectopic pregnancy. Lancet. 2005 Aug 13-19; 366(9485): 583-91.*

- *CDC Ectopic Pregnancy Surveillance. http://www.cdc.gov/mmwr/ preview/mmwrhtml/00014677.htm*

#27

The radiology resident refuses to do the pelvic ultrasound you ordered to rule out an ectopic because the hCG on your patient is 100, and he states that women can not rupture an ectopic pregnancy when the beta is that low.

Is this statement true or false?

    A. True

    B. False

#27

Answer: B

The radiologist's statement is false. A single hCG level cannot rule in or rule out an ectopic pregnancy. A hCG in a patient who presents to the ED with abdominal pain or vaginal bleeding with a hCG < 1500 are less likely to have a normal IUP. A beta hCG < 1500 in these patients more than doubles the odds of having an ectopic pregnancy. Women can rupture an ectopic pregnancy with an hCG at any level. The risk of ectopic pregnancy is in fact increased when the likelihood of a normal IUP is low. Therefore, transvaginal ultrasound should be performed in women at risk for ectopic pregnancy, regardless of the hCG level.

• Kohn MA, et al. Beta-human chorionic gonadotropin levels and the likelihood of ectopic pregnancy in emergency department patients with abdominal pain or vaginal bleeding. Acad Emerg Med. 2003 Feb;10(2): 119-26. full text

#28

Regarding venous thromboembolism and pregnancy, which of the following is TRUE?

A. 30% of isolated episodes of pulmonary embolism are associated with silent deep-vein thrombosis (DVT).

B. The majority of cases of pulmonary embolism occur in the first trimester.

C. DVTs occur more commonly in the right leg, rather than the left leg.

D. Ultrasound reliably detects DVT in the iliac vein.

Amy Kaji

#28
Answer: A

Approximately 30% of episodes of pulmonary embolism are associated with silent deep-vein thrombosis. In patients with an DVT, the frequency of silent pulmonary embolism ranges from 40 to 50%.

Venous thromboembolism is both more common and more complex to diagnose in patients who are pregnant than in those who are not pregnant. The incidence of venous thromboembolism is estimated at 0.76 to 1.72 per 1000 pregnancies, which is four times greater than in the nonpregnant population. A meta-analysis showed that two thirds of cases of deep-vein thrombosis occurred in the antepartum period and were distributed relatively equally among all three trimesters. There is a predisposition for deep-vein thrombosis to occur in the left leg (approximately 70 to 90% of cases), possibly because of the compressive effects from the right iliac artery on the the left iliac vein.

Although compression ultrasonography is the test of choice in pregnant patients, iliac DVTs are are not easily detected by ultrasonography. Isolated iliac-vein DVTs may present as abdominal pain, back pain, and swelling of the entire leg.

- Marik PE, Plante LA. *Thromboembolism and Pregnancy. N Engl J Med. 2008 Nov 6; 359(19): 2025-33.*

#29

Regarding thromboembolism and pregnancy, which of the following statements is TRUE?

- A. Compression ultrasonography is accurate for isolated calf vein thrombosis.

- B. Magnetic resonance direct thrombus imaging has a high sensitivity and specificity for the diagnosis of iliac-vein thrombosis.

- C. Warfarin is the preferred agent for anticoagulation in pregnancy.

- D. If your patient is pregnant and is on a low-molecular weight heparin (LMWH), then factor Xa should be monitored and accordingly adjusted.

- E. Bed rest is the recommended treatment modality.

#29

Answer: B

Compression ultrasonography is a noninvasive test with a sensitivity of 97% and a specificity of 94% for the diagnosis of symptomatic, proximal deep-vein thrombosis but is less accurate for isolated calf and iliac vein thrombosis. Magnetic resonance direct thrombus imaging has a high sensitivity and specificity for the diagnosis of iliac vein thrombosis.

In pregnancy, the D-dimer level increases through the pregnancy and can be used in combination with imaging since a positive D-dimer is often difficult to interpret.

Chan et al. showed that a negative D-dimer in the first and second trimesters had a negative predictive value of 100%; the sensitivity and specificity of a positive test were 100% and 60%, respectively. A negative D-dimer test may be helpful, whereas a positive D-dimer test should mandate a lower extremity compression ultrasound.

The treatment and prophylaxis of venous thromboembolism in pregnancy should not involve warfarin. There is significant fetal harm such as facial abnormalities and limb growth defects, especially within the first 6-9 weeks of gestation. Unfractionated heparin or low-molecular-weight heparin is the preferred anticoagulant during pregnancy associated DVT.

In all patients on LMWH, monitoring anti–factor Xa activity and dose adjustments are not required except in patients at the extremes of body weight and those with altered renal function. Bed rest is generally not recommended for patients with deep-vein thrombosis, unless there are complications such as phlegmasia.

. *LLSA 2011: Marik PE, Plante LA. Thromboembolism and Pregnancy. N Eng J Med. 2008: 359(19): 2025-2033. full text*

. *Chan WS, et al. A red blood cell agglutination D-dimer test to exclude deep venous thrombosis in pregnancy. Ann Intern Med. Ann Intern Med. 2007 Aug 7; 147(3): 165-70. full text*

. *Bagaria S, Bagaria V. B. Strategies for Diagnosis and Prevention of Venous Thromboembolism during Pregnancy. J Pregnancy. 2011; 1-7.*

#30

Regarding thromboembolism and pregnancy, which of the following statements is TRUE?

A. Treatment with low-molecular-weight heparin may be resumed within 12 hours after delivery in the absence of persistent bleeding.

B. Low-molecular-weight heparin or warfarin is recommended for at least 6 weeks postpartum and for a total of at least 6 months.

C. Women who have had a thromboembolic event have a much higher risk of a recurrent episode during pregnancy than women without such a history.

D. Patients presenting with pulmonary embolism in late pregnancy should be treated with supplemental oxygen (to achieve an oxygen saturation of >95%) and intravenous heparin with transfer to a center with maternal-fetal medicine.

E. The incidence of pulmonary embolism is reported to be higher after cesarean section than after vaginal delivery.

F. All of the above

#30

Answer: F

Current guidelines from the American Society of Regional Anesthesia and Pain Medicine recommend that LMWH for the the treatment of pulmonary embolism in pregnancy be resumed within 12 hours after delivery if there is no bleeding. Furthermore, they recommend that anticoagulation with either LMWH or warfarin be continued for at least 6 weeks postpartum and for a total treatment time of at least 6 months.

Patients presenting with pulmonary embolism in late pregnancy should have oxygen saturation maintained at >95% and anticoagulation with heparin. Recommendations also favor transfer to a center with maternal-fetal medicine and cardiothoracic surgery for patients with a large clot burden.

A temporary vena caval filter is a possible treatment option since there is a high risk of a recurrent PE in pregnant women. Although thromboembolism after cesarean section is uncommon, the incidence is higher than vaginal delivery. Venous thromboembolism after cesarean section is uncommon but is reported to be higher than after vaginal delivery, by a factor of 2.5 to 20. The incidence of fatal pulmonary embolism is increased by a factor of 10.

• Horlocker TT, et al. Executive summary: regional anesthesia in the patient receiving antithrombotic or thrombolytic therapy: American Society of Regional Anesthesia and Pain Medicine Evidence-Based Guidelines (Third Edition). Reg Anesth Pain Med. Jan-Feb 2010; 35(1): 102-5 full text

#31

The most common symptom of placenta previa is:

A. Painful uterine contractions

B. Signs of fetal distress

C. Painful vaginal bleeding

D. Painless vaginal bleeding

E. Hemodynamic instability of the mom

#31

Answer D

Painless vaginal bleeding is the most common symptom of placenta previa. It occurs due the the placental implantation over the cervical os and bleeding is more often present during the second trimester. In the ED, speculum examination of the vagina and cervix should only be performed in consultation with OBGYN. Other external signs of bleeding can be examined such as hemorrhoids and vaginal lacerations.

- *Rosen's Emergency Medicine - Concepts and Clinical Practice. 8th edition. 2013. Chapter 178: Acute Complications of Pregnancy. 2289-2290.*

Amy Kaji

#32

An intrauterine pregnancy can be diagnosed by sonographic findings in the following correct order of appearance:

A. Fetal pole, double gestational sac, double ring sign, and fetal heart rate activity

B. Double gestational sac, fetal pole, double ring sign, and fetal heart rate activity

C. Double ring sign, double gestational sac, intrauterine fetal pole, and intrauterine fetal heart activity

#32

Answer: C

The development of ultrasound findings of an intrauterine pregnancy occur in the following order: the double ring sign, the double gestational sac, the intrauterine fetal pole, and intrauterine fetal heart activity. There is not a definitive hCG level that correlates with the ability to visualize a IUP on ultrasound, and only a yolk sac confirms an IUP.

In general, transvaginal ultrasound can identify an intrauterine gestational yolk sac at 5 weeks (estimated hCG of 1800 IU/liter), while fetal heart motion can be detected with the transvaginal ultrasound at 6 weeks' gestation (estimated hCG of 6770 IU/L).

- *Rosen's Emergency Medicine - Concepts and Clinical Practice. 8th edition. 2013. Chapter 177: General Approach to the Pregnant Patient. 2275.*

#33

You are seeing a patient who is Rh (Anti-D) negative woman who is pregnant at 10 weeks. Anti-D immuno-globulin (RhoGAM) administration would be indicated if the father is Rh positive or his status is unknown during all of the following scenarios EXCEPT:

A. Threatened miscarriage

B. Spontaneous miscarriage

C. Surgery for ectopic pregnancy

D. Amniocentesis

E. Speculum exam

#33
Answer: E

Rh immunization in pregnancy occurs when an Rh negative woman is exposed to Rh-positive fetal blood. A small number of fetal cells enter the maternal circulation spontaneously throughout pregnancy but the maternal immune system is only triggered by significant loads of fetal cells, which can occur during the 3rd trimester and at delivery. Sensitization occurs in up to 15% of Rh negative women carrying Rh-positive fetuses. To prevent this, anti-D immunoglobulin (RhoGAM) is routinely administered to Rh-negative mothers if the father is Rh-positive or his status is unknown, at approximately the 29th week of gestation. Transplacental hemorrhage can also occur during uterine manipulation, threatened miscarriage, spontaneous miscarriage, surgery for ectopic pregnancy, and amniocentesis. A dose of 50 micrograms can be used if the patient is at less than 12 week and after 12 weeks a 300 microgram dose should be given. The half life of immunoglobulin is 24 days and it needs to be administered within 72 hours of a sensitization event to prevent antibody development.

- *Bowman J. Rh-immunoglobulin: Rh prophylaxis. Best Pract Res Clin Haematol. 2006; 19(1): 27-34.*

- *SmartEM - Threatened Ab: Knowledge is Power. http://smartem.org/podcasts/threatened-ab-knowledge-power*

#34

A 29 yo female presents with vaginal spotting for the last 5 days associated with left lower quadrant abdominal pain. You suspect possible ectopic pregnancy. TRUE statements about this entity include which of the following?

(Choose three answers.)

A. Incidence of ectopic pregnancy has decreased over the last several decades.

B. 90% of women who have ectopic pregnancies have a risk factor for an ectopic.

C. A single serum hCG value neither identifies the presence of an intrauterine or ectopic pregnancy nor predicts rupture, but it can serve as a surrogate marker for gestational age.

D. "Discriminatory zone" (when a sonogram should detect an IUP) hCG values have been reported to be between 1500 to 3000 mIU.

E. In 8 to 31% of women in whom ectopic pregnancy is suspected, the initial ultrasound does not show a pregnancy in either the uterus or in the fallopian tubes.

#34
Answer: C, D, and E

The incidence of ectopic pregnancy increased by a factor of six between 1970 and 1992, but it has since remained stable. No newer data is available. The associated mortality has decreased markedly to 0.5 deaths per 1000, because of early diagnosis and treatment before rupture. Damage to the fallopian tubes from PID, prior tubal surgery, or a previous ectopic pregnancy is strongly associated with an increased risk of ectopic. However, half of all women who receive a diagnosis of an ectopic do NOT have any risk factors. The risk of recurrence of ectopic is 10% among patients with one previous ectopic and at least 25% among women with 2 or more previous ectopics. The ultrasound may be non-diagnostic because the gestational sac may not have developed in an early IUP, and an early ectopic may be too small for visualization.

• Barnhart KT. Ectopic pregnancy. N Engl J Med. 2009 Jul 23; 361(4): 379-87.

• Kamwendo F, Forslin L, Bodin L, Danielsson D. Epidemiology of ectopic pregnancy during a 28 year period and the role of pelvic inflammatory disease. Sex Transm Infect. 2000; 76(1): 28.

Amy Kaji

#35

A 29 yo female presents with vaginal spotting for the last 5 days associated with left lower quadrant abdominal pain. You suspect possible ectopic pregnancy. TRUE statements about DIAGNOSING this entity include which of the following?

A. Serial measurement of hCG can help distinguish potentially viable IUPs from an ectopic.

B. 50% of women with ectopics present with increasing hCG levels and 50% present with decreasing hCG levels.

C. In women who have decreasing hCG levels, serial hCG should be performed until hCG is no longer detectable in the serum (this may take 6 weeks).

D. Sensitivity and specificity of progesterone level is not sufficiently high to rule in or rule out an ectopic pregnancy.

E. The accuracy of ultrasound varies according to the serum hCG level.

F. All of the above

#35

Answer: F

All of the statements are true. Approximately 99% of viable IUPs are associated with an increase in hCG levels of at least 53% in 2 days (note that this is slower than the doubling that is commonly taught). Although statement B is true, 71% of women with ectopics have serial serum hCG values that increase more slowly than would be expected with a viable IUP or decrease more slowly than would be expected with a miscarriage. Regarding accuracy of ultrasound, in one study, when the hCG value was < 1500IU/L, the positive predictive value of ultrasound for an IUP was only 80% and that for an ectopic was only 60%.

- *LLSA 2012: Barnhart KT. Ectopic pregnancy. N Engl J Med. 2009 Jul 23;361(4):379-87.*

#36

Which of the following treatments should be offered to a woman presenting 72 hours after a rape?

A. Medroxyprogesterone

B. Levonorgestrel

C. Mifepristone

D. Pitocin

E. Copper IUD

#36

Answer: B

The reported risk of pregnancy in a woman of childbearing age after rape is 5% and progestin-only emergency contraception (levonorgestrel 1.5 mg), which is administered within 120 hours after unprotected intercourse has been shown to be 98.5% effective in preventing pregnancy. Unlike mifepristone (RU486), levonorgestrel does not cause an abortion and there is no evidence of it harming a fetus if the woman is pregnant. It may cause nausea, vomiting, abdominal pain, and vaginal bleeding.

- *Linden JA. Care of the adult patient after sexual assault. N Engl J Med. 2011 Sep 1; 365(9): 834-41.*

#37

True or False: some ectopic pregnancies resolve spontaneously without medical (methotrexate) or surgical therapy.

    A. True

    B. False

#37

Answer: A

True. Some ectopic pregnancies resolve spontaneously without therapy but this should not be the default assumption. Although case series suggested rates of resolution as high as 70%, these rates are derived from selected cases of early tubal gestations with hCG values < 1000 mIU that were already decreasing. Women who are offered the option of expectant management (e.g., watchful waiting) must be informed of the potential risk of tubal rupture despite decreasing hCG values. Close coordination is required with OB/GYN and the decision for expectant management should not be made by the ED physician.

- *LLSA 2012: Barnhart KT. Ectopic pregnancy. N Engl J Med. 2009 Jul 23; 361(4): 379-87.*

OPHTHALMOLOGY

#1

Your patient sustained an orbital blowout fracture of the floor and medial wall after an assault. He has diplopia on upward gaze from inferior rectus muscle entrapment and anesthesia over the anteromedial cheek and upper lip from stretch on the infraorbital nerve. Your patient previously had intact vision, but he now complains of decreased visual acuity, severe pain, and is noted to have proptosis. What should you do?

A. Administer prednisolone eye drops.

B. Administer pilocarpine eye drops.

C. Administer tetracaine eye drops to ease the pain.

D. Drain the orbital hematoma by performing a lateral canthotomy.

E. Place a patch on the eye.

#1

Answer: D

Injury to the orbit, particularly fractures, can cause a retro-orbital hematoma, which as it increases in size, will lead to proptosis. The increasing retro-orbital pressure will also limit flow to the retinal artery leading to visual loss. In this case, a lateral canthotomy should be performed to drain the retro-orbital blood.

• *Roberts and Hedges' Clinical Procedures in Emergency Medicine. 6th edition. 2013. Chapter 62: Ophthalmologic, Otolaryngologic, and Dental Procedures. 1293-1295.*

#2

You are seeing a 3 week old infant in whom you are considering dacryocystitis vs. congenital nasolacrimal duct obstruction (CNLDO). All of the following would be signs consistent with CNLDO, EXCEPT:

A. Excessive tear lake

B. Mucoid discharge

C. Crusting or stickiness of the eye

D. Swollen and red eye

E. Tear overflow

#2

Answer: D

With CNLDO, there may be excessive tearing or discharge that is produced by the lacrimal sac. However, the conjunctivae are clear and there should be no signs of infection. In contrast, dacryocystitis is characterized by erythematous and swollen skin over the lacrimal sac and purulent drainage from the punctum. Fever may be present and periorbital and orbital cellulitis may develop as a complication of dacryocystitis.

. *Pinar-Sueiro S, et al. Dacryocystitis: Systematic Approach to Diagnosis and Therapy. Curr Infect Dis Rep. 2012 Jan 29. full text*

#3

You suspect dacryocystitis in a 2 week old neonate. All of the following should be performed, EXCEPT:

A. Discharge with outpatient antibiotics.

B. Administration of antibiotics that cover strepto-coccus and staphylococcus.

C. Immediate consultation with ophthalmology.

D. Continued monitoring for development of sepsis.

E. Culture of purulent drainage.

#3

Answer: A

In the infant who is 1 month or younger with dacryocyst-itis, admission for IV antibiotics is required. Dacryocyst-itis in a neonate is associated with significant number of systemic complications and requires inpatient admission. The most dreaded complication is development of meningitis and sespsis. Immediate consultation with an ophthalmologist is also required.

• Pinar-Sueiro S, et al. Dacryocystitis: Systematic Approach to Diagnosis and Therapy. Curr Infect Dis Rep. 2012 Jan 29. full text

#4

You are seeing a patient with super glue (cyanoacrylate glue) in his right eye. Which of the following should NOT be performed?

A. Pain medication, as needed

B. If the glue is adherent to the cornea, then it should be treated like a corneal abrasion with antibiotics and mydriatic agents.

C. Reexamination of the eye in 24-48 hours

D. Surgical trimming of the eyelashes to forcefully open the eye

#4

Answer: D

Typically, eyelids are permitted to separate on their own, which will occur over a course of 1 to 4 days. If needed, erythromycin eye ointment or bacitracin ointment can be used to facilitate eyelid separation. However, the lashes should not be pulled out or surgically removed.

- *Roberts and Hedges' Clinical Procedures in Emergency Medicine. 6th edition. 2013. Chapter 63: Otolaryngologic Procedures. 1317.*

#5

Which of the following will cause a relative afferent pupillary defect (RAPD)?

A. Optic nerve damage

B. Retinal detachment

C. Vitreous hemorrhage

D. Traumatic mydriasis

E. All of the above

#5

Answer: E

A RAPD suggests any of the following: efferent third nerve damage, glaucoma, iris incarceration, massive internal derangement of the eye (trauma to the eye so severe that the light pathway is disrupted and is significantly decreased), optic chiasm or tract damage, optic nerve damage, retinal detachment, traumatic mydriasis, or vitreous hemorrhage. To test for a RAPD in the traumatized eye, the physician should observe the pupil symmetry and size of the non traumatized or unaffected eye while swinging a bright light from eye to eye. When the light strikes the unaffected eye, the pupil constricts. When the light strikes the affected eye, the pupil of the unaffected eye paradoxically dilates.

• *Rosen's Emergency Medicine - Concepts and Clinical Practice. 8th edition. 2013. Chapter 71: Ophthalmology. 913-914.*

#6

Absence of a red reflex or inability to visualize the fundus suggests all of the following EXCEPT:

A. Optic nerve damage

B. Cataract

C. Significant hyphema

D. Lens rupture

E. Significant vitreous hemorrhage

#6

Answer: A

Absence of a red reflex or inability to visualize the fundus suggests an issue with passage of light from the anterior to the posterior chamber. Diseases can include cataract, hyphema, lens rupture, obstructing mass, and vitreous hemorrhage.

- *Rosen's Emergency Medicine - Concepts and Clinical Practice. 8th edition. 2013. Chapter 71: Ophthalmology. 915-916.*

#7

A normal intraocular pressure (IOP) ranges from 10 to 20 mm Hg. An elevation greater than 22 mmHg classically may occur in all of the following conditions EXCEPT:

    A. Acute glaucoma

    B. Hyphema

    C. Suprachoroidal hemorrhage

    D. Retrobulbar hemorrhage

    E. Globe penetration

#7

Answer: E

An elevated intraocular pressure > 22 can be seen any of the following:

1. Acute glaucoma
2. Hyphema
3. Suprachoroidal hemorrhage
4. Retrobulbar hemorrhage.

IOP measurement is contraindicated if there is a suspected open globe. When the pressure is less than 5 mm Hg, penetration of the globe should be suspected.

- *Rosen's Emergency Medicine - Concepts and Clinical Practice. 8th edition. 2013. Chapter 71: Ophthalmology. 910-915.*

#8

The most common cause of persistent tearing, infection, and discharge in the pediatric population is:

A. Nasolacrimal duct obstruction

B. Conjunctivitis

C. Uveitis

D. Lid abnormalities, such as ectropion and entropion

E. Corneal abnormalities, such as abrasions and ulcers

#8

Answer: A

Nasolacrimal duct obstruction is the most common cause of persistent tearing, infection, and ocular discharge in children. The other causes range from mild self-limited conditions to ocular emergencies that can also cause tearing, infection, and discharge in children.

• *Rosen's Emergency Medicine - Concepts and Clinical Practice. 8th edition. 2013. Chapter 71: Ophthalmology. 923.*

#9

True statements about endophthalmitis include all of the following EXCEPT:

    A. It can affect the vitreous of the eye.

    B. It can affect the aqueous humor of the eye.

    C. It can be caused by CMV and other herpes viruses.

    D. It is an ophthalmologic emergency.

    E. Cataract surgery and glaucoma surgery are risk factors for bacterial endophthalmitis.

#9

Answer: C

Endophthalmitis refers to a bacterial or fungal infection of the vitreous or aqueous humor of the eye. In contrast, viruses tend to infect the retina or uvea, causing retinitis and uveitis. The acute presentation of endophthalmitis is a ophthalmologic emergency and requires an ophthalmology consult and prompt intravenous and intraocular antibiotics. Endophthalmitis is also a complication of ocular surgery and globe trauma.

Rosen's Emergency Medicine - Concepts and Clinical Practice. 8th edition. 2013. Chapter 71: Ophthalmology. 918.

#10

You are seeing a patient with traumatic hyphema. The cornerstone of management is to prevent which of the following TWO complications?

A. Conjunctivitis

B. Uveitis

C. Intraocular hypertension

D. Rebleeding

E. Blepharitis

#10

Answer: C and D

The main focus of treating a traumatic hyphema is prevention of elevated intraocular pressure. Secondary hemorrhage can lead to vision loss and is more common in large hyphemas or in patients with underlying coagulopathies. The intraocular pressure should be frequently monitored with close ophthalmology follow-up. Recommendations are for patients to limit activity and maintain head elevation. Consultation with ophthalmology is required since patients will need very close follow-up for repeat pressure measurements.

- *Rosen's Emergency Medicine - Concepts and Clinical Practice. 8th edition. 2013. Chapter 71: Ophthalmology. 913-915.*

- *ERCast - Hyphema: http://blog.ercast.org/hyphema/*

#11

Which of the following is NOT consistent with globe rupture?

    A. Increased intraocular pressure

    B. Markedly decreased visual acuity

    C. Increased anterior chamber depth

    D. Seidel's sign

    E. Eccentric pupil

#11

Answer: A

An open globe should be ruled out prior to applying pressure to the eye to perform tonometry. In the presence of an open globe, Seidel's sign may be seen when fluorescein is added to the eye. Depending on the degree of laceration to the globe there may also be an accompanied irregular pupil, decreased visual acuity and a low intraocular pressure. In general, the tonometry to measure intraocular pressure can be deferred until ophthalmologic consultation if an open globe is highly suspect.

Physical findings of globe rupture include:

1. Markedly decreased visual acuity
2. Eccentric pupil
3. Increased anterior chamber depth
4. Low intraocular pressure
5. Extrusion of vitreous
6. External prolapse of the uvea or other internal ocular structures
7. Tenting of the cornea or sclera at the site of globe puncture
8. Seidel's sign, in which fluorescein will flow in a tear drop pattern away from the puncture site

- *Rosen's Emergency Medicine - Concepts and Clinical Practice. 8th edition. 2013. Chapter 71: Ophthalmology. 915-916.*

#12

Regarding periorbital and orbital cellulitis all of the following are true EXCEPT:

A. Periorbital cellulitis is an infection lying posterior to the orbital septum.

B. Periorbital cellulitis is associated with eyelid swelling, discoloration of the orbital skin, conjunctival injection.

C. Orbital cellulitis tends to have similar but more severe symptoms than periorbital cellulitis and also include proptosis, pain, and decreased ocular mobility.

D. Changes in vision, extraocular movements, and pupillary findings are normal in preseptal cellulitis.

E. If orbital cellulitis is suspected, a CT of the orbit is the most useful aid to determine retro-orbital involvement.

#12

Answer A

Periorbital cellulitis is an infection lying anterior to the orbital septum. Differentiation between preseptal vs. orbital cellulitis is an important clinical decision that affects management. Both tend to be associated with swelling and pain, but orbital cellulitis is more commonly associated with proptosis and limited ocular mobility. Sinusitis is the leading cause in up to 80% of cases. Treatment of preseptal cellulitis is outpatient broadspectrum anti-staphylococcal agent with daily follow up. Orbital cellulitis treatment includes ophthalmologic evaluation in the ED, hospitalization, IV antibiotics and in some cases, surgery for debridement.

- Rosen's Emergency Medicine - Concepts and Clinical Practice. 8th edition. 2013. Chapter 71: Ophthalmology. 920-921.

#13

You are seeing a 5 yo patient with a hyphema after he sustained blunt trauma to the eye. Which of the following are reasonable indications for admission?

A. Grade 3 or 4 hyphema

B. Presence of a bleeding dyscrasia (sickle cell disease)

C. If the patient has an elevated intraocular pressure

D. Suspected globe rupture

E. Suspected child abuse

F. All of the above

#13

Answer: F

Several observational studies suggest that most patients can safely receive treatment for hyphema in the outpatient setting. Inpatient management is recommended for patients with:

- Multiple ocular or facial injuries
- Suspected abuse
- Coagulopathy
- Sickle cell disease
- Intraocular hypertension
- Globe injury
- Large hyphemas (filling of 50% or more of the anterior chamber).

Patients must be able to avoid activity, and follow-up closely with an ophthalmologist. All patients should have an eye shield placed, head maintained upright at 30 degrees, and have reversal of any underlying coagulopathy.

Hyphema grades as percentage of anterior chamber filled with blood:

Grade 1: <33%

Grade 2: 33-50%

Grade 3: 50-90%

Grade 4: 90-100%

- Brandt MT, Haug RH. Traumatic hyphema: a comprehensive review. J Oral Maxillofac Surg. 2001 Dec;59(12): 1462-70.

#14

You are seeing a 35 year old female who presents with 1 day of redness of the right eye, without any associated pain or visual loss. There is some increased tearing. You are entertaining the diagnosis of episcleritis vs. scleritis. Which of the following statements about episcleritis is FALSE?

A. 70% of episcleritis patients are women.

B. Patients with episcleritis usually complain of the abrupt onset of redness, irritation, and watering of the eye.

C. Vision is not affected by episcleritis, and approximately one-half of cases are bilateral.

D. Episcleritis is not sight-threatening and is self-limiting.

E. Episcleritis is more often associated with systemic diseases, rather than scleritis.

#14

Answer: E

The episclera is vascularized connective tissue that lies beneath the conjunctiva but superficial to the sclera. Episcleritis, is characterized by redness of the episclera and is painless. Scleritis, however, presents with intense pain, photophobia and a dark reddish-purple discoloration.

Episcleritis is a benign disorder, while scleritis can destroy the cornea and uvea. Although it is possible to have isolated scleritis, there is a strong association with rheumatoid arthritis or Wegener's granulomatosis. Scleritis can be treated with steroids or immunosuppressants in coordination with ophthalmology.

• *Rosen's Emergency Medicine - Concepts and Clinical Practice. 8th edition. 2013. Chapter 118: Systemic Lupus Erythematosus and the Vasculitides. 1537.*

• *Rosen's Emergency Medicine- Concepts and Clinical Practice. 8th edition. 2013. Chapter 22: Red and Painful Eye. 190.*

#15

True or False: Both pterygium and pinguecula are associated with increased exposure to ultraviolet light.

    A. True

    B. False

#15

Answer A

True. A pterygium is a wedge-shaped area of conjunctival tissue that extends onto the cornea. Pinguecula is a whitish-yellow raised area of conjunctiva next to the cornea that unlike pterygium does not extend onto the cornea. Both are associated with UV light exposure and are usually asymptomatic except for some associated irritation or redness. Treatment is supportive with protection against dry eyes using artificial tears and UV protection by wearing sunglasses.

- *Threlfall TJ, English DR. Sun exposure and pterygium of the eye: a dose-response curve. Am J Ophthalmol. Sep 1999; 128(3): 280-7.*

#16

A 62 yo woman presents with a 1 week history of a large floater in the left eye associated with "light flashes" in the left peripheral field. She reports a "cloud that moves around her visual field" and though she can see well enough to watch TV, her vision is decreased. TRUE statements about this patient presentation include which of the following?

(Choose three answers.)

A. The most likely diagnosis of patients who report acute onset floaters and flashes is posterior vitreous detachment (PVD).

B. PVD is more common in the younger population.

C. Risk factors for PVD includes myopia, trauma, and intraocular inflammation.

D. All floaters and/or flashes represent ocular problems.

E. Prevalence of retinal tears among patients with flashes but no floaters is almost identical to those who present with floaters but no flashes.

#16

Answer: A, C, and E

Posterior vitreous detachment involves separation of the posterior vitreous from the retina as degeneration and loss of tissue volume occurs. It increases in occurrence with increasing age. The prevalence increases from 24% in adults aged 50-59 to 87% among those aged 80-89. Not all floaters and flashes represent ocular problems, and non-ocular causes can usually be differentiated by a careful history. Migraine headaches, occipital lobe disorders, and postural hypotension can all cause floaters and flashes. Either flashers or floaters can signify the beginning of a retinal tear.

- *Hollands H, et al. Acute-Onset Floaters and Flashes Is. This Patient at Risk for Retinal Detachment? JAMA. 2009 Nov 25; 302(20): 2243-9. full text*

#17

Chalazion is often confused with a hordeolum. Which of the following is TRUE regarding hordeolum and chalazion?

    A. Internal hordeolum involves the meibomian glands.

    B. External hordeolum involves the glands of Zeis or Moll at the base of the eyelashes.

    C. A chalazion is a firm, non-tender lump that arises from obstruction of a meibomian gland.

    D. All of the above

#17

Answer: D

Blockage of the meibomian glands can form either a chalazion or internal hordeolum. If a chronic granulomatous reaction with cyst formation develops, then a chalazion is formed. If an acute inflammation or abscess develops, then an internal hordeolum is formed. Management of hordeolum and chalazion are usually conservative. Lid hygiene, warm compresses, and topical antibiotic ointments are usually adequate.

- *Rosen's Emergency Medicine - Concepts and Clinical Practice. 8th edition. 2013. Chapter 22: Red and Painful Eye. 193.*

#18

You suspect that a patient you are seeing has anterior uveitis or iritis. Which of the following statements about uveitis is FALSE?

A. Patients may report pain, tearing, photophobia, and decreased visual acuity.

B. There may be ciliary flush.

C. The pupil may appear miotic and distorted.

D. Topical analgesics will significantly ameliorate the pain.

E. Consensual photophobia is common.

#18

Answer: D

Key diagnostic features of anterior uveitis are a miotic pupil, ciliary flush, and the findings of cell and flare in the anterior chamber. Uveitis is inflammation of any of the pigmented vascular structures of the eye, which include the iris, ciliary body, and choroid. A pathognomonic finding for iritis is consensual photophobia.

Anterior uveitis is often associated with systemic diseases such as rheumatoid arthritis, sarcoidosis, Behcet disease, Sjogren syndrome, ankylosing spondylitis, inflammatory bowel disease, Reiter's syndrome, and infectious diseases (TB, toxo, herpes, CMV, syphilis, AIDS, and Lyme disease).

Topical analgesics do not significantly ameliorate the pain of anterior uveitis. Intraocular pressure may be decreased due to compromised aqueous production. Ophthalmologic referral is key so that topical cycloplegics and steroids can be administered and titrated to symptoms.

- Agrawal R, et al. Current approach in diagnosis and management of anterior uveitis. Indian J Ophthalmol. 2010 Jan-Feb; 58(1): 11–19. full text

#19

You are seeing a patient who complains of painless visual loss. As you are thinking of the differential diagnosis, which of the following can most likely be ELIMINATED because the patient has no pain?

(Choose two answers.)

    A. Optic neuritis

    B. Uveitis

    C. CRAO (central retinal artery occlusion)

    D. CRVO (central retinal vein occlusion

    E. Amaurosis fugax

#19

Answer: A and B

CRAO, CRVO, and amaurosis fugax cause painless visual loss. Optic neuritis is an inflammatory disorder and is often the initial manifestation of MS. Most patients have pain with eye movements. Typically, there is unilateral involvement and an afferent pupillary defect, and elevation of the optic disc may be seen on fundoscopic exam. Uveitis is inflammation of the iris, ciliary body, or choroid, and most patients present with conjunctival injection, pain, photophobia and blurred vision.

- *Rosen's Emergency Medicine - Concepts and Clinical Practice. 8th edition. 2013. Chapter 71: Ophthalmology. 923-927.*

#20

You are seeing a patient with binocular diplopia due to an acute 3rd nerve palsy. TRUE statements about this entity include which of the following?

(Choose three answers.)

A. The two most common causes are an aneurysm of the posterior communicating artery and diabetes.

B. Diplopia occurs in all directions of gaze except for medial gaze of the affected side.

C. Most patients with a space-occupying lesions (aneurysm or mass) present with a ptosis, diplopia, and headache.

D. Ischemia from diabetes usually spares the pupil, because the pupillary-constrictor fibers have a dual blood supply from the core and sheath of the 3rd cranial nerve.

#20

Answer: A, C, and D

The 3rd nerve innervates the muscles of the eyelid and all external ocular muscles, except the superior oblique and the lateral rectus. Parasympathetic fibers run along the external surface of the 3rd nerve. If there is a compressive force on the the nerve, ischemia will cause decrease in parasympathetic activity causing unopposed sympathetics dilating the eye. This creates the classic "blown" pupil. Because a complete 3rd nerve palsy innervates the levator palpebrae, paralysis will cause ptosis. The eyelid can still be tightly shut via the 7th cranial nerve. Diplopia occurs in all directions of gaze except for lateral gaze of the affected side as the lateral rectus is intact.

- *Capo H, et al. Evolution of Oculomotor Nerve Palsies. J Clin Neuroo-phthalmol. 1992 Mar; 12(1): 21-5.*

#21

True or False: the most common cause of a 4ᵗʰ nerve palsy is from aneurysmal disease.

    A. True

    B. False

#21

Answer: B

Isolated 4th nerve (trochlear) palsies are most commonly caused by trauma but can also occur from diabetes or mass effect. Aneurysmal compression is rare. The 4th nerve innervates the superior oblique and paralysis causes diplopia when the patient looks down and away from the affected eye. Patients may describe difficulty descending stairs or reading a book.

- *Rosen's Emergency Medicine - Concepts and Clinical Practice. 8th edition. 2013. Chapter 21: Diplopia. 197-198.*

#22

True or False: There is a strong association with idio-pathic intracranial hypertension and 6th cranial nerve (CN) palsy.

    A. True

    B. False

#22

Answer: A

The 6th nerve is easily tested with lateral gaze. The nerve innervates the lateral rectus causing the patient to have difficulty with lateral gaze. Aneurysmal disease is uncommon. There is a strong association with 6th nerve palsy and elevated intracranial pressure. This should always prompt neuroimaging. CN 6 is theorized to be easily affected by elevated intracranial pressure due to its long circuitous route through the cavernous sinus.

- *Rosen's Emergency Medicine - Concepts and Clinical Practice. 8th edition. 2013. Chapter 21: Diplopia. 197-198.*

#23

You are treating a patient with a unilateral painful eye with redness and photophobia, and you suspect traumatic iritis. In your medical decision making, you state: "no peri-limbic sparing, cell and flare present." This means:

A. The area surrounding the cornea is more red than the other conjunctiva, and the anterior chamber is cloudy.

B. The area surrounding the cornea is less red than the other conjunctiva and the anterior chamber is cloudy.

C. The area surrounding the cornea is more red than the other conjunctiva and the anterior chamber is not cloudy.

D. The area surrounding the cornea is less red than the other conjunctiva and the anterior chamber is not cloudy.

#23

Answer: A

Peri-limbic sparing indicates that the uvea is not involved and is common in conjunctivitis. The opposite is true for ciliary flush. Ciliary flush occurs due to ciliary body inflammation. Uveitis, and iritis, cause ciliary flush. Uveal inflammation also typically causes protein and WBCs to cloud the anterior chamber producing cell and flare. Patients with traumatic iritis also have consensual photophobia.

. *Rosen's Emergency Medicine - Concepts and Clinical Practice. 8th edition. 2013. Chapter 71: Ophthalmology. 926.*

. *Andy Neill - CFN Eye Anatomy http://vimeo.com/115529933*

#24

In the patient that you suspect has optic neuritis, you should do which of the following:

(Choose two answers.)

A. Start prednisone orally and discharge the patient home.

B. Start prednisone orally and admit the patient.

C. Start IV methylprednisolone and admit the patient.

D. Consider obtaining an MRI of the brain with and without contrast.

E. Perform a lumbar puncture immediately.

#24

Answer: C and D

An MRI of brain with gadolinium can help confirm the diagnosis of MS as well as demyelinating optic neuritis. Lumbar puncture is not useful for diagnosis of optic neuritis and should be reserved for patients who also have meningitis or encephalitis as part of the differential diagnosis. Patients with optic neuritis and MS will have a nonspecific lumbar puncture that may show elevated protein or lymphocytes. Treatment with intravenous methylprednisolone for children and adults with either severe vision loss or two or more white matter lesions on MRI is recommended. Treatment is associated with a more rapid recovery of vision but does not impact long-term visual function.

Oral prednisone does not affect short or long-term visual outcomes in acute optic neuritis and may be associated with an increased risk of recurrent optic neuritis.

• *Rosen's Emergency Medicine - Concepts and Clinical Practice. 8th edition. 2013. Chapter 71: Ophthalmology. 926.*

• *Optic Neuritis Study Group. The clinical profile of optic neuritis. Experience of the Optic Neuritis Treatment Trial. Optic Neuritis Study Group. Arch Ophthalmol. 1991; 109(12): 1673-8.*

#25

A patient is sent to you from an outside ED with acute monocular visual loss and you suspect optic neuritis. Features that would be consistent with optic neuritis include all of the following EXCEPT:

A. Pain with extraocular movement

B. An afferent pupillary defect

C. Papillitis on fundoscopic exam

D. Corneal edema

E. Demyelinating lesions seen on MRI of the brain

#25

Answer: D

Optic neuritis is an inflammatory, demyelinating condition affecting the optic nerve that causes acute, usually monocular, visual loss. There is a high association with multiple sclerosis (MS). The Optic Neuritis Treatment Trial (ONTT) showed that 90% patients experience loss of central visual acuity as a presenting problem along with pain with extraocular movements. Patients may also have an afferent pupillary defect. The characteristic findings on MRI for MS are demyelinating lesions. Papillitis with hyperemia, blurring of disk margins, and distended veins, are seen in one-third of patients with optic neuritis. Corneal edema is a finding more likely in postoperative patients after a cataract removal.

• *Rosen's Emergency Medicine - Concepts and Clinical Practice. 8th edition. 2013. Chapter 71: Ophthalmology. 926.*

• *Optic Neuritis Study Group. The clinical profile of optic neuritis. Experience of the Optic Neuritis Treatment Trial. Optic Neuritis Study Group. Arch Ophthalmol. 1991 Dec; 109(12): 1673-8.*

ORTHOPEDICS

Amy Kaji

#1

You are seeing a patient with a tense lower leg, and you are concerned about compartment syndrome. The patient has sustained a tibia-fibular fracture and he has plantar paresthesia, weakness of toe flexion, and pain with passive extension of the toes. Which of the following compartment is most likely to be involved?

A. Anterior compartment

B. Lateral compartment

C. Deep posterior compartment

D. Superficial posterior compartment

E. Medial compartment

#1
Answer: C

The lower leg is a frequent area for acute compartment syndrome (ACS). There are four compartments to the lower leg:

1. Anterior
2. Lateral
3. Deep posterior
4. Superficial posterior

Anterior Compartment: The anterior compartment of the leg is the most common compartment involved. It contains:

1. Extensor muscles of the foot
2. Anterior tibial artery
3. Deep peroneal nerve.

Early on, patients will experience loss of sensation between the first and second toes and decreased dorsiflexion strength. As complete deep peroneal nerve involvement occurs, patients develop foot drop.

Lateral Compartment:

1. Controls foot eversion
2. Contributes to plantar flexion
3. Contains the the peroneal artery
4. Contains the superficial peroneal nerve
5. Contains the proximal portion of the deep peroneal nerve.

Increased pressure in the lateral compartment can cause a proximal deep peroneal nerve deficit, which will be evident by weakness with dorsiflexion and inversion of the foot. Similar to lateral compartment involvement patients will have loss of sensation in the first web space.

As the superficial peroneal nerve becomes involved, sensory loss will occur over the anterior lower leg and dorsum of the foot.

Superficial Posterior Compartment:

1. Contains the major muscles of plantar flexion
2. Does not contain any major arteries or nerves travel in this compartment.

The superficial posterior compartment of the leg is the least likely to develop compartment syndrome.

Deep Posterior Compartment:

1. Contributes to plantar flexion
2. Contains the posterior tibial artery
3. Contains the peroneal artery
4. Contains the tibial nerve

Involvement of the deep posterior compartment will manifest as weakness with toe flexion and pain with passive extension of the toes and plantar paresthesia.

. *Rosen's Emergency Medicine - Concepts and Clinical Practice. 8th edition. 2013. Chapter 49: General Principles of Orthopedic Injuries. 519-25.*

#2

You are seeing a 5 year old with a supracondylar humerus fracture, and you suspect compartment syndrome of the forearm. Which of the following is the LEAST likely physical finding?

A. Decreased wrist extension

B. Decreased flexion of the distal interphalangeal joints of the index and middle finger

C. Decreased flexion of the interphalangeal joint of the thumb

D. Decreased flexion of the distal interphalangeal joints of the ring and little finger

#2

Answer: A

The forearm has four compartments:

1. Deep volar compartments
2. Superficial volar compartment
3. Dorsal compartment
4. Lateral compartment

The volar compartments contains the digital flexors and the dorsal compartment contains the digital extensors. Both volar compartments are at high risk for developing ACS.

Supracondylar fractures in children and distal radius fractures in adults are the most common injuries associated with forearm ACS. The deep volar compartment is at risk of developing the greatest pressure with ACS and thus the flexor digitorum profundus (responsible for distal interphalangeal joint flexion) and the flexor pollicis longus (responsible for interphalangeal joint flexion of the thumb) muscles are most often affected.

The wrist flexors and extensors are rarely involved.

• *Rosen's Emergency Medicine - Concepts and Clinical Practice. 8th edition. 2013. Chapter 49: General Principles of Orthopedic Injuries. 519-525.*

#3

A 42 year old male painter who is right hand dominant presents with left hand pain after he was using a paint gun containing paint thinner that went off trajectory and into the palmar aspect of his left hand and his middle finger. All of the following are true statements about high-pressure injection injuries EXCEPT:

A. The type of material is the most important element in determining the subsequent morbidity.

B. The amount of material injected determines tissue distention, compression, and mechanical distortion of blood flow.

C. The clinical appearance is determined by the time elapsed between injury and presentation.

D. Pain control is optimally delivered via a digital nerve block.

E. ED treatment includes elevation of the extremity, administration of broad-spectrum antibiotics, tetanus prophylaxis, and preparation for surgery.

#3

Answer: D

Pain control may be provided through opiates. Performing a digital nerve block is contraindicated because adding the extra volume can further accentuate a compartment syndrome. Increasing the temperature of the extremity via a warm compresses increases blood flow and compromise tissue perfusion even more due to the increased pressure. Immediate surgical consultation is the treatment of choice.

- *Rosen's Emergency Medicine - Concepts and Clinical Practice. 8th edition. 2013. Chapter 50: Hand. 562-563.*

#4

A 23 year old basketball player presents with what appears to be a painful right ring finger after he "jammed" his finger into the ball. Regarding mallet finger injuries, which of the following is FALSE?

A. The mechanism of injury is often sudden forceful flexion of an extended finger when an object, such as a ball, strikes the tip of the finger.

B. There are three types of injury: type 1 tendon rupture (no fracture), type 2 tendon avulsion with a small bone fragment, and type 3 tendon avulsion with a large bone avulsion.

C. The DIP, PIP, and MCP should be immobilized for 6 weeks.

D. Only 30-40% of patients regain normal function of the DIP joint after treatment.

#4

Answer: C

The primary goal of treatment is the maintenance of distal interphalangeal joint extension. Treatment of type 1 and 2 injuries is nonoperative. Immobilization can be accomplished with either a volar or a dorsal splint made from a variety of materials, including aluminum and plastic. The DIP joint is immobilized in slight hyperextension for 6 to 8 weeks, but the PIP and MCP joints are allowed to move freely. Definitive treatment of a type 3 injury is controversial. Some authors recommend operative repair; others recommend conservative management with uninterrupted splinting of the digit. The prognosis of mallet fingers is marginal by any method; only 30 to 40% regain normal function in the DIP joint after treatment.

- *Rosen's Emergency Medicine - Concepts and Clinical Practice. 8th edition. 2013. Chapter 50: Hand. 557-558.*

#5

You are treating a right-hand dominant patient for a paronychia. All of the following statements about paronychia are true, EXCEPT:

A. A paronychia begins as a cellulitis, but an abscess may form.

B. E. coli is the most common isolate, followed by anaerobes.

C. Atypical mycobacteria and Candida albicans should be considered as etiologic agents in chronic cases.

D. In the early cellulitis phase, management consists of frequent warm soaks, elevation, and administration of antibiotics.

E. When the area becomes fluctuant, drainage can be accomplished by advancing a no. 11 blade scalpel or an 18-gauge needle parallel to the nail and under the eponychium at the site of maximal swelling.

#5

Answer: B

Staph aureus is the most common isolate, followed by streptococci. Paronychias in children are often caused by anaerobes, and it is believed that this is due to nail biting and finger sucking. Atypical mycobacteria and candida albicans should be considered as etiologic agents in chronic cases. A well-known complication of even a properly drained paronychia is osteomyelitis of the distal phalanx.

- *Rosen's Emergency Medicine - Concepts and Clinical Practice. 8th edition. 2013. Chapter 50: Hand. 565-566.*

#6

A 14-year old boy was skateboarding down a hill when he had to turn abruptly to avoid a car pulling out of an alley. He states he heard a "crack", and was immediately unable to ambulate. On exam, he has swelling over the anterior distal leg and ankle. He has no pain or tenderness around the knee, medial malleolus, proximal fibula, or foot. What is the most likely injury:

A. Maisonneuve fracture

B. Lisfranc fracture-dislocation

C. Ça-ne-fait-rien deformity

D. Tillaux fracture

Amy Kaji

#6

Answer: D

A Tillaux fracture is a Salter-Harris type III fracture of the lateral distal tibia, seen almost exclusively in adolescents. The predisposing pathophysiology seems to result from asymmetric physeal closure: the adolescent's mid portion of the distal tibial physis fuses before the lateral portion. A compression-torque stress on the joint causes an avulsion of the lateral epiphysis. Plain films may not show the fracture, and CT may be required to make the diagnosis. Fragments displaced more than 2 mm are generally treated surgically.

A Maisonneuve fracture is the combination of a medial malleolar fracture with an oblique fracture of the proximal fibula (forces transmitted through the interosseous ligament). They most often require open reduction and internal fixation (ORIF).

A Lisfranc deformity refers to injury along the tarsometatarsal joint. If not apparent on physical exam or standard radiographs, weight-bearing films may be used to accentuate the dislocation. CT can be used if there is high suspicion. Treatment is ORIF versus percutaneous pinning.

The "Ça-ne-fait-rien" deformity has yet to be described in the medical literature, because we made it up!

• *Wheeless III, CR. Duke Orthopedics. Tillaux Fracture. Wheeless Textbook of Orthopaedics. http://www.wheelessonline.com/ortho/tillaux_fracture*

• *Wheeless III, CR. Duke Orthopedics. Lisfranc's Fracture / TarsoMetatarsal Injuries. Wheeless Textbook of Orthopaedics. http://www.wheelessonline.com/ortho/lisfrancs_fracture_tarsometatarsal_injuries*

#7

Regarding felons, which of the following statements is FALSE?

    A. A felon is an infection of the pulp of the distal finger or thumb.

    B. It differs from other types of subcutaneous abscesses because of the presence of multiple vertical septa that divide the pulp into small fascial compartments.

    C. The incision should be made along the radial aspect of the index, middle, and ring fingers, and the ulnar aspects of the thumb and little finger, avoiding the pincher surfaces.

    D. Any incision that is made too deep can injure the flexor tendon sheath.

    E. Untreated, the expanding abscess can extend toward the phalanx, producing an osteitis or osteomyelitis.

#7

Answer: C

Most felons can be drained by a single lateral incision. The incision should be made along the **ulnar aspect of the index, middle, and ring fingers** and along the **radial aspects of the thumb and little finger (non-pressure bearing side of digit).** The incision is begun approximately 0.5 cm distal to the DIP joint with careful avoidance of the neurovascular bundle of the fingertip. The incision is extended to the free edge of the nail. The wound should be irrigated extensively. Most felons are treated empirically with anti-staphylococcal oral antibiotics for at least 5 days pending culture results.

- *Rosen's Emergency Medicine - Concepts and Clinical Practice. 8th edition. 2013. Chapter 50: Hand. 566.*

#8

Regarding flexor tenosynovitis, all of the following statements are true, EXCEPT:

A. All patients with flexor tenosynovitis require hospital admission and consultation with a hand surgeon.

B. The four cardinal signs of acute flexor tenosynovitis include: 1) tenderness along the course of the flexor tendon; 2) symmetric swelling of the finger; 3) pain with passive extension; and 4) an extended posture of the finger.

C. Early recognition and treatment are necessary because elevated pressure within the enclosure of the tendon sheath can occlude the blood flow resulting in necrosis.

D. Disseminated gonorrhea should be considered in all sexually active individuals, especially if there is no apparent traumatic etiology of the infection.

E. Infections are usually caused by penetrating trauma to the sheath, but they occasionally result from hematogenous spread.

F. The most commonly isolated organism is Staph aureus.

#8

Answer: B

Four cardinal signs of acute flexor tenosynovitis (Kanavel's Signs) are usually present to help distinguish tenosynovitis from other soft tissue infections of the hand:

1. Tenderness along the tendon sheath
2. Symmetric swelling of the finger
3. Pain with passive extension
4. A flexed posture of the finger.

The third sign is often the most important and earliest finding.

- *Rosen's Emergency Medicine - Concepts and Clinical Practice. 8th edition. 2013. Chapter 50: Hand. 566-567.*

#9

Regarding carpal instability injuries, commonly sustained after a fall onto an outstretched hand, which of the following statements is FALSE?

A. A scapholunate dissociation results in a characteristic widening of the scapholunate joint on the posteroanterior and stress views.

B. A perilunate dislocation demonstrates the capitate in the appropriate position relative to a dorsally displaced lunate.

C. A lunate dislocation results in a characteristic triangular appearance of the lunate on the posteroanterior view because of the rotation of the lunate in a volar direction. This is known as the "piece of pie" sign.

D. In a lunate dislocation, a lateral view of the wrist will show the lunate appearing as a cup tipped forward ("spilled teacup sign").

E. Complications of carpal dislocation injuries include median nerve injury and chronic carpal instability.

#9

Answer: B

In a perilunate dislocation, the lunate remains in position relative to the distal radius, and the capitate is dorsally dislocated. The posteroanterior view shows overlap of the distal and proximal carpal rows and may show an associated scaphoid fracture or subluxation.

- *Rosen's Emergency Medicine - Concepts and Clinical Practice. 8th edition. 2013. Chapter 50: Hand. 580-582.*

#10

You are reviewing some elbow X-rays of patients. All of the following are true, EXCEPT:

A. The radiographically normal elbow has a narrow strip of lucency anteriorly and posteriorly.

B. Normally, fat surrounding the proximal elbow joint is hidden in the concavity of the olecranon and coronoid fossa.

C. When the anterior humeral line transects the anterior third of the capitellum or passes entirely anterior to it, you should suspect a supracondylar fracture.

D. When a posterior fat pad is seen in the setting of trauma, in adults, a radial head fracture is implied, and in children, a supracondylar fracture is the probable underlying injury.

E. The fat pad sign may be absent with a fracture if the injury is severe enough to have ruptured the capsule.

#10

Answer: A

The radiographically normal elbow has only an anterior fat pad, visible as a narrow lucency. A posterior fat pad should NOT be visible. In the setting of a fracture, the anterior fat pad also is altered by swelling, becoming more prominent and taking the shape of a sail from a boat. In the setting of trauma, posterior fat pad sign is associated with up to 90% of intra-articular injuries.

- *Rosen's Emergency Medicine - Concepts and Clinical Practice. 8th edition. 2013. Chapter 50: Hand. 598-601.*

#11

Regarding plantar fasciitis, which of the following statements is FALSE?

A. It is caused by degeneration and inflammation of the fascia that extends from the calcaneal tuberosity to the metatarsal heads.

B. Physical examination may demonstrate reproduction of pain with passive dorsiflexion of the ankle or toes.

C. Treatment is focused on relaxing the tension on the fascia.

D. One treatment modality is the use of plantar-flexion night splints.

E. Rest, ice, stretching of the gastrocnemius muscle, arch taping, use of orthotics, administration of anti-inflammatory drugs, wearing proper shoes, and surgery are all recommended treatments.

F. Patients will have heel pain while standing on their toes.

#11

Answer: D

Treatment is focused on elongating the plantar fascia. Dorsiflexion night splints may be used. The premise of night splints is to keep the foot in a slightly dorsiflexed position to minimize plantar-fascial shortening. All of the other statements are true.

•   *Rosen's Emergency Medicine - Concepts and Clinical Practice. 8th edition. 2013. Chapter 58: Ankle and Foot. 748.*

•   *Bolgla L, Malone T. Plantar Fasciitis and the windlass mechanism: a biomechanical link to clinical practice. J Athl Train. 2004 Jan; 39(1): 77-82. full text*

#12

Which of the following statements about perilunate and lunate dislocations is FALSE?

A. Lunate and perilunate dislocations are best seen on the lateral radiographic view.

B. Suspect a lunate or perilunate dislocation if a straight line does not pass through the centers of the distal radius, lunate, and capitate.

C. With a perilunate dislocation, the capitate has alignment with the radius, but the lunate is volarly rotated and displaced.

D. On the PA view in a lunate dislocation, the rotated lunate takes on a triangular shape known as the "piece of pie" sign.

E. ED management of both lunate and perilunate dislocations includes immobilizing the wrist in the neutral position in a volar splint and hand surgeon consultation.

#12

Answer: C

With a perilunate dislocation, the lateral radiograph demonstrates disarticulation of the capitolunate joint. The capitate is dorsally displaced and the lunate should appear in its normal position. With a lunate dislocation, the capitate aligns in a straight line with the radius, but the lunate is volarly rotated and displaced. The displacement of the lunate has a "spilled teacup" appearance.

- *Rosen's Emergency Medicine - Concepts and Clinical Practice. 8th edition. 2013. Chapter 50: Hand. 580-582.*

#13

Regarding radial styloid fractures, which of the following is TRUE?

A. A direct blow along the radial side of the wrist can produce an oblique or transverse fracture of the radial styloid.

B. Intra-articular radial styloid fractures are known as a Chauffeur's or a Hutchinsons' fracture.

C. Displaced fractures can produce carpal instability, resulting in scapholunate or other carpal dislocations.

D. ORIF is frequently required for even minimal displacement.

E. All of the above

#13

Answer: E

All of the statements are true. The major carpal ligaments of the radial side of the wrist insert on the radial styloid. Thus, displaced fractures can produce carpal instability resulting in scapholunate or other carpal dislocations.

. *Distal Radius Fracture http://www.orthobullets.com/ trauma/1027/distal-radius-fractures*

#14

In a patient with an ulnar shaft fracture, what other associated injury should your examine the patient for?

A. Radial styloid fracture

B. Ulnar styloid fracture

C. Scaphoid fracture

D. Radial head dislocation

E. Metacarpal dislocation

#14

Answer: D

Ulnar shaft fractures result most often from direct blows to the forearm, most commonly to ward off an assailant's blow (nightstick fracture). Nondisplaced, non-angulated fractures are immobilized using anterior-posterior splints, with the elbow in 90 degrees of flexion and the forearm neutral.

Patients with these injuries should be examined carefully for evidence of associated radial head dislocation (Monteggia fracture-dislocation). Usually, there is pain and tenderness to palpation at the elbow, and the radial head may be palpated in a posterior or anterior location. In adults, these fracture-dislocations are treated with ORIF, whereas in children, adequate closed reduction may be achieved.

• *Rosen's Emergency Medicine - Concepts and Clinical Practice. 8th edition. 2013. Chapter 51: Wrist and Forearm. 591-592.*

#15

True statements about spinal stenosis include all of the following EXCEPT:

A. Pain is relieved by standing and spinal extension.

B. It is due to narrowing of the spinal canal that may occur at single or multiple spinal levels and is associated with radiculopathy or claudication.

C. Symptoms usually begin in the fifth or sixth decade.

D. Pain is relieved by rest and forward flexion.

E. Classic symptom includes pseudoclaudication, which is pain of the lateral legs that occurs with walking, and is relieved with rest.

#15

Answer: A

Symptoms of spinal stenosis include low back pain aggravated by prolonged standing and spinal extension with pain relieved by rest and forward flexion. Seen in 60% of patients, pseudoclaudication is the classic symptom where pain of the lateral legs occurs with walking and is relieved with rest. It is termed pseudoclaudication because it is caused by neurologic compression, rather than arterial insufficiency.

• *Rosen's Emergency Medicine - Concepts and Clinical Practice. 8th edition. 2013. Chapter 54: Musculoskeletal Back Pain. 646.*

#16

Regarding hip dislocations, which of the following is FALSE?

A. Posterior dislocations optimally need reduction within 6 hours to minimize the risk for avascular necrosis, and the reduction should be attempted in the ED.

B. Anterior hip dislocations occur most commonly from a direct blow to the abducted hip.

C. The posteriorly dislocated hip can be reduced by flexing the hip, creating traction in line with the deformity, and applying internal and external rotation.

D. Anterior hip dislocations are more common than posterior hip dislocations.

E. Careful neurovascular examination is mandatory after an anterior dislocation, owing to the risk of arterial damage and venous thrombosis.

#16

Answer: D

Posterior hip dislocations are more common than anterior dislocations and result from force applied to a flexed knee and hip (when the knee hits the dashboard during a motor vehicle crash). The hip is forcefully adducted and flexed while it is pushed posteriorly. On examination in a posterior hip dislocation, the limb is flexed, adducted, and internally rotated with limb shortening. Anterior dislocations most commonly result from a direct blow to the abducted hip.

- *Roberts and Hedges' Clinical Procedures in Emergency Medicine. 6th edition. 2013. Chapter 49: Management of Common Dislocations. 985-989.*

#17

A 13 year old girl who is a soccer player presents with bilateral knee pain (right greater than left). On exam, she has tenderness to palpation at the distal aspect of her tibial tubercle. There is no direct joint or patellar tenderness and she has a steady gait without hip or ankle pain. The anterior drawer, posterior drawer, and McMurray's tests are all negative. She denies any fever, weight loss, or pain at night, but she states the pain has forced her to intermittently sit out of soccer practice this past week. What is NOT true about this syndrome?

A. More commonly occurs in boys 10-15 years old.

B. Treatment is conservative and symptomatic with ice, activity modification, NSAIDs, quadriceps strengthening.

C. Even mild pain is an absolute contraindication to sports and the patient should not return until pain free.

D. Recovery usually occurs within weeks but in some cases not until the growth plate is completely closed.

E. This condition is due to apophyseal injury to the tibial tubercle in adolescents.

#17

Answer: C

This case describes Osgood-Schlatter Syndrome, which occurs more commonly in boys. However, this trend is changing as girls 8-13 yrs of age are increasingly involved in competitive sports. Mild pain during activity is not an absolute contraindication to participation, but with more severe symptoms, the risk of avulsion of the tibial tubercle must be considered. It is important to evaluate for a tibial tubercle avulsion on X-ray.

. *Rosen's Emergency Medicine - Concepts and Clinical Practice. 8th edition. 2013. Chapter 176: Musculoskeletal Disorders. 2269.*

#18

Regarding carpal dislocations and injuries, which of the following statements is FALSE?

A. Carpal stability is based on the lunate as the central anchor for the proximal and distal carpal rows.

B. Disruption of the first row of carpal bones on an AP radiograph is suggestive of a lunate dislocation.

C. Disruption of the second row of carpal bones on an AP radiograph is suggests a perilunate dislocation.

D. Normally, the lunate appears to be triangular on an AP view, and when it appears to be quadrangular, it suggests a lunate dislocation.

E. Kienbock disease, or avascular necrosis of the lunate, may follow lunate dislocations, even if there is successful reduction in the ED.

#18

Answer: D

Carpal stability is based on the lunate as the central anchor for the proximal and distal carpal rows. The lunate is opposed to the radius, and the capitate rests within the lunate cup. The proximal row of carpals is connected by interosseous ligaments. Carpal stress is translated to all bones. Ligamentous injury results in a spectrum of injuries, including lunate and perilunate dislocations.

On a normal AP wrist X-ray, two arcs should be identified. The first arc consists of the radiocarpal row. Disruption is suggestive of a lunate dislocation. The second arc consists of the midcarpal row. Disruption of this arc is suggestive of a perilunate dislocation. The appearance of the lunate is important on the AP view. Normally, the lunate is quadrangular, however, with lunate dislocations, it becomes triangular. This may be an additional clue to dislocation.

On the lateral view, visualize linear bone alignment of the radius, lunate, and capitate. The lunate should lie within the radius cup and the capitate should align with lunate. Loss of this linear arrangement suggest lunate or perilunate dislocation. Soft-tissue complications include carpal ligament disruption, which results in carpal instability. Kienbock disease, or avascular necrosis of the lunate, may occur following lunate dislocations, even if there is successful reduction in the ED.

• Rosen's Emergency Medicine - Concepts and Clinical Practice. 8th edition. 2013. Chapter 51: Wrist and Forearm. 580-582.

#19

An eight-year old boy is brought in by his mother for arm pain. He has had this pain before, but it became much worse yesterday after he played his first baseball game. There is no history of blunt trauma. The child complains of pain in his arm and elbow. On exam, he has tenderness to palpation over the medial humeral condyle, with normal strength, sensation, pulses and no ecchymosis or gross deformity. The most likely cause of his pain is:

A. Acromioclavicular (AC) separation

B. Shoulder dislocation

C. Radial head subluxation

D. Valgus stress on the affected joint

#19

Answer: D

Little leaguer's elbow is a chronic overuse injury of the medial humeral condyle caused by repetitive valgus stress, resulting in osseous damage of the elbow. This injury can be seen in baseball players (pitchers and non-pitchers alike), racquetball and football players. X-rays may show hypertrophy or separation of the medial humeral condyle. Treatment consists of rest until symptoms are completely resolved, followed by "re-training" in proper throwing mechanics.

Shoulder dislocation is uncommon in children less than 10 years old. However, if an adolescent does dislocate the shoulder, re-dislocation rates are relatively high.

Radial head subluxation, or Nursemaid's elbow, generally occurs in children 1-3 years old. The immature radial head becomes entrapped distal to the annular ligament after longitudinal traction. The hyperpronation method of relocation has a higher success rate (97.5%) than the supination-flexion method (86%).

- *Rosen's Emergency Medicine - Concepts and Clinical Practice. 8th edition. 2013. Chapter 52: Humerus and Elbow. 610-611.*

- *Macias CG, et al. A comparison of supination/flexion to hyperpronation in the reduction of radial head subluxations. Pediatrics. 1998 Jul; 102(1):e10. full text*

#20
What is considered a normal compartment pressure?

    A. 15-20 mm Hg

    B. 20-25 mm Hg

    C. 0-5 mm Hg

    D. 25-30 mm Hg

    E. 30-35 mm Hg

#20

Answer: C

The normal pressure of a tissue compartment falls between 0 and 8 mmHg. Acute Compartment Syndrome (ACS) may develop when pressure exceeds 35 mm Hg or is within 35 mm Hg of diastolic blood pressure. Sustained compartment pressures > 20 mm Hg increase the risk of peripheral nerve injury in patients with hypotension or peripheral vascular disease, ACS can develop at lower pressures. A single normal compartment pressure reading, does NOT rule out ACS. Repeated measurements depending on symptoms are necessary to ensure the diagnosis is not missed.

ACS develops soon after trauma and is more common in long bone fractures of the lower leg or forearm. ACS may also occur in patients without trauma and is reported as a complications of coagulopathy with compartmental bleeding, animal envenomations and bites, extravasation of IV fluids and contrast, IV drug abuse, and prolonged limb compression.

- *Rosen's Emergency Medicine - Concepts and Clinical Practice. 8th edition. 2013. Chapter 49: General Principles of Orthopedic Injuries. 521-523.*

#21

You are seeing a patient with hip pain and you are considering septic arthritis as part of your differential diagnosis. Risk factors for septic hip arthritis include which of the following?

A. Prosthetic joint

B. Age > 80

C. Diabetes

D. IV drug abuse

E. Previous intra-articular steroid injection

F. All of the above

#21

Answer: F

Predisposing factors for septic arthritis in adults were identified in a 2007 systematic review that included a total of 6242 patients with acutely painful joints; 653 (10%) had septic arthritis and the predisposing factors and the associated value as predictors (reflected by the estimated positive likelihood ratios [+LR]) are summarized as follows:

1. Age greater than 80 years
2. Diabetes mellitus
3. Rheumatoid arthritis
4. Prosthetic joint
5. Recent joint surgery
6. Skin infection
7. Cutaneous ulcers
8. IV drug abuse
9. Alcoholism
10. Previous intra-articular corticosteroid injection.

Each of these factors appears to have a modest impact on the risk of septic arthritis, however, combinations of independent risk factors lead to substantially increased risk. As an example, acute joint pain in the presence of a joint prosthesis and evidence of skin infection is associated with a +LR of 15 (95% CI 8.1-28). However, septic arthritis does not appear to occur more often in patients with HIV infection than in other patients.

- Mathews CJ, Kingsley G, Field M, et al. Management of septic arthritis: a systematic review. Ann Rheum Dis. 2007; 66(4): 440-5.

#22

You are seeing a 3 year old male patient with sickle cell anemia in whom you suspect osteomyelitis of the foot and tibia. All of the following statements are true about this diagnosis and its associated complications, EXCEPT:

A. The annual incidence in sickle cell patients is approximately 0.36%.

B. The prevalence of osteomyelitis after foot puncture wounds in diabetics can be as great as 40%.

C. Mortality rates are low.

D. DVT is not a known complication of osteomyelitis involving the long bones.

E. Complications include spread of infection to associated soft tissues or joints; evolution to chronic infection, amputation of the involved extremity, and sepsis.

Amy Kaji

#22

Answer: D

Up to 30% of pediatric patients with long-bone osteo-myelitis may develop deep venous thrombosis (DVT). The development of DVT may also be a marker for disseminated infection. Organisms involved in osteo-myelitis in include staphylococcus pneumococcus and salmonella species. Pending cultures antibiotics should be selected to treat these organisms. In addition to dir-ect wounds at the involved extremity, hematogenous spread should be suspected and thorough evaluation for distal sources of infection should be ruled out.

- *Calhoun JH, Manring MM. Adult osteomyelitis. Infect Dis Clin North Am. 2005 Dec; 19(4): 765-86.*

- *Concia E, et al. Osteomyelitis: clinical update for practical guide-lines. Nucl Med Commun. Aug 2006; 27(8): 645-60.*

284

#23

Thorough knowledge of the anatomy and functions of the hand is required for proper diagnosis and treatment of hand injuries. Use of proper terminology prevents confusion that may compromise the care of patients with hand injuries. All of the following statements about terminology, anatomy, and function are true EXCEPT:

A. The proper names of the 5 digits beginning radially are thumb, index finger, long or middle finger, ring finger, and little finger.

B. There are intrinsic and extrinsic muscles of the hand. Extrinsic muscles course the forearm and insert into hand while intrinsic muscles arise and end in the hand.

C. The blood supply to the hand is derived from the ulnar and radial arteries.

D. The radial nerve sends intrinsic motor branches to the hand.

E. Lateral motion of the hand is described as radial deviation when the palm is supinated or ulnar deviation when the palm is pronated.

#23

Answer: D

The median, ulnar, and radial nerves supply the sensory innervation to the hand. The median nerve passes through the carpal tunnel before entering the hand and then provides motor innervation to the three thenar muscles and the first and second lumbricals. The ulnar nerve provides motor innervation to the hypothenar muscles, the two ulnar lumbricals, the adductor pollicis, and all of the interosseous muscles. The radial nerve does not provide motor branches to the intrinsic muscles of the hand. All of the rest of the statements are true.

- *Rosen's Emergency Medicine - Concepts and Clinical Practice. 8th edition. 2013. Chapter 50: Hand. 542-543.*

#24

You are seeing a patient with a patellar dislocation. TRUE statements about this orthopedic injury include which of the following?

(Choose three answers.)

A. Patellar dislocations most commonly occur in the seventh and eighth decades.

B. Males are affected more than females.

C. Manual reduction is necessary if spontaneous reduction has not occurred.

D. Reduction of a medial dislocation can be accomplished by flexing the hips to relax the quadriceps then slowly extending the knee while medial pressure is applied to the lateral aspect of the dislocated patella.

E. After reduction and complete evaluation, the knee should be placed in a patella stabilizing brace or in a knee immobilizer until a brace may be obtained.

#24
Answer: C, D and E

Patellar dislocation occurs most often in the second and third decades of life with girls more affect than boys. The most common mechanism is a twisting movement on a fixed knee. Direct trauma can also cause a dislocation. The lateral dislocation is most common although a medial or intraarticular dislocation can also occur. For a lateral dislocation manual reduction is easily performed in the emergency department. It is often more comfortable for the patient if done under procedural sedation. The knee will be held in a flexed position and the knee is slowly extended with medially directed pressure applied from the lateral aspect. The patella will "pop" back into the tibiofemoral tract and the patient will have return of knee mobility. A knee immobilizer will provide comfort to the patient after the reduction.

• *Roberts and Hedges' Clinical Procedures in Emergency Medicine. 6th edition. 2013. Chapter 49: Management of Common Dislocations. 993.*

• *WikEM - Patellar Disslocation http://www.wikem.org/wiki/ Patella_Dislocation*

#25

You are seeing a patient with a humeral shaft fracture. Which of the following statements is FALSE regarding humeral shaft fractures?

   A. Most humeral shaft fractures warrant operative repair.

   B. Initial evaluation should involve inspection of skin integrity, neurovascular function, deformity, shortening, etc.

   C. If the shoulder is thought to be involved, then shoulder radiographs should include a scapular-Y or axillary view to assure that there is no associated dislocation.

   D. Nonoperative management of humeral shaft fractures often involve immobilization in a sugar-tong splint.

   E. The most common neurologic complication of a humeral shaft fracture is radial nerve injury.

Amy Kaji

#25

Answer: A

Initial evaluation of the patient with an upper arm injury includes inspection for laceration, neurovascular deficits, deformities, and then plain radiographs. Shoulder radiographs should include an axillary or scapular-Y confirming that the humeral head is not dislocated. Most (70 to 80%) of humerus shaft fractures can be treated without surgical intervention. Initial immobilization is usually accomplished with a coaptation (sugar-tong) splint or a sling. For oblique and spiral fractures that require moderate traction, a collar and cuff sling can be used. All open fractures should have operative exploration for vascular injuries.

Emergent orthopedic consultation is required for articular injuries, and concomitant forearm fractures (floating elbow injuries), pathologic fractures and in polytrauma. Distal shaft fractures (Holstein Lewis fractures) have a very high association with radial nerve injuries. Radial nerve ischemia and nonunion are the more common complications . These complications can occur in 10% of fractures. Most radial nerve injuries will self resolve in a few months; however, orthopedic referral is important. Nonunion occurs more often with transverse and comminuted fractures.

• Rosen's Emergency Medicine - Concepts and Clinical Practice. 8th edition. 2013. Chapter 52: Humerus and Elbow. 601-604.

#26

You are seeing a patient with an elbow dislocation. All of the following statements are true EXCEPT:

(Choose two answers.)

A. One third of elbow dislocations are associated with fractures of the elbow.

B. A fall onto an extended abducted arm is the mechanism of injury seen in posterior dislocations of the elbow.

C. Anterior dislocations account for the majority of elbow dislocations.

D. Dislocations occur more commonly in children because of the instability of their ligaments.

E. A strong blow to the posterior aspect of a flexed elbow may result in anterior dislocation of the elbow.

F. Anterior elbow dislocations and any open fracture can disrupt the brachial artery and median nerve.

#26

Answer: C and D

Dislocations occur more commonly in adults, since the same force in children more often results in a supracondylar fracture of the distal humerus. Posterior dislocations account for most elbow dislocations. Closed posterior dislocations are not commonly associated with neurovascular injury.

• *Rosen's Emergency Medicine - Concepts and Clinical Practice. 8th edition. 2013. Chapter 52: Humerus and Elbow. 612-613.*

#27

You are now seeing a patient in whom you suspect a knee dislocation. All of the following statements about this disease are true EXCEPT:

A. Posterior dislocations have a increased risk of causing a popliteal artery injury.

B. Anterior dislocations are caused by hyperextension.

C. Twenty to thirty percent of all knee dislocations are complicated further by open joint injury.

D. Coexistent peroneal nerve injury occurs in 25-35% of patients and must be ruled out.

E. An ankle-brachial index between 0.95 and 1.2 is abnormal and would warrant further imaging (duplex ultrasound or CT angiography).

#27

Answer: E

The ankle-brachial index (ABI) compares the pressure of an arm to a leg as a screening tool for lower limb ischemia. The measurement is performed with a doppler and compares the highest doppler pulse detection of the posterior tibial or dorsalis pedis artery to the brachial pulse. The ankle doppler pressure is divided by the brachial doppler pressure to calculate the index. An ABI less than 0.9 indicate an abnormal result and should prompt further vascular imaging/assessment.

Anterior knee dislocations are caused by severe knee hyperextension and require at least 30 degrees of hyperextension before dislocation.

Posterior knee dislocations occur with a posterior directed force to the proximal tibia and usually occur with a motor vehicle accident dashboard impact. The majority of dislocations are posterior and there is a risk of popliteal artery injury. If there are no obvious vascular injuries but the ABI is < 0.9, then surgical consult is necessary and vascular imaging should be performed.

Traditionally, arteriography was performed, but increasingly, duplex ultrasonography (100% sensitivity and 97% specificity for clinically significant arterial injury), or CT angiography (95-100% sensitivity and 97-98% specificity for clinically significant arterial injury) is being used. Peroneal nerve function should also be assessed since there can be as high as a 35% rate of injury and is manifested by loss of sensation in the first toe webspace with decreased foot dorsiflexion.

• Henrichs. A. A Review of Knee Dislocations. J Athl Train. 2004 Oct-Dec; 39(4): 365–369. full text

#28

Regarding proximal tibial fractures, which of the following is TRUE?

(Choose three answers.)

A. Medial plateau fractures are more common than lateral plateau fractures.

B. Lateral tibial plateau fractures usually result from a direct blow.

C. Avulsion of the anterior tibial spine usually occurs in the adult population, rather than in the pediatric/adolescent population.

D. If the suspicion is high for a tibial plateau fracture but is not seen on plain radiograph, then MRI or CT is indicated.

E. Avulsion of the anterior tibial spine often results in a significant effusion.

#28

Answer: B, D, and E

Proximal tibial fractures are classified for management purposes into those that affect the medial or lateral tibial plateau and fractures of the intercondylar notch. Tibial plateau fractures most commonly involve the lateral plateau after a direct blow that produces a strong force to the lateral knee. Often when X-rays are negative but the patient has significant pain, a CT or MRI will help visualize the injury. CT will better define a fracture but does not visualize the meniscal or ligamentous structures.

Medial tibial plateau fractures require a higher force due to the increased joint strength. Due to to the force required for the injury, if the fracture involves the medial aspect there is also lateral plateau injury as well.

Avulsion of the anterior tibial spine is more common in children while adults with a similar mechanism will often experience an anterior cruciate ligament (ACL). Both injuries will show large knee effusions and may require outpatient MRI imaging.

• *Rosen's Emergency Medicine - Concepts and Clinical Practice. 8th edition. 2013. Chapter 57: Knee and Lower Leg. 706-708.*

#29

You are seeing a patient in whom you suspect an ulnar collateral ligament injury (gamekeeper's or skier's thumb). Which of the following statements is FALSE regarding this entity?

A. The patient may have decreased pincer grasp and ability for opposition of the thumb to the index finger.

B. Varus stress testing determines the stability of the ligament.

C. The patient may complain of pain over the metacarpophalangeal (MP) joint.

D. X-rays are usually normal (there may be bony avulsion at the base of the insertion of the ligament at the phalanx).

E. Referral to an orthopedist or hand surgeon is indicated for patients who have a bony fragment on X-ray that is more than 1 mm displaced or involves greater than 10% of the articular surface.

#29

Answer: B

Valgus stress testing determines the integrity of the ulnar collateral ligament. A comparison should be made to the stability of the opposite thumb. The ligament can be strained (pain without abnormal movement), partially torn (pain and increased movement), or completely disrupted. Specifically, an incomplete rupture is characterized by less than 30 degrees of laxity or less than 15 degrees more laxity than in the non-injured thumb. A complete rupture is characterized by more than 30 degrees or more than 15 degrees more laxity than in the non-injured thumb.

PA and lateral X-rays of the thumb are indicated in patients with suspected gamekeeper's thumb to identify bony avulsion of the ulnar collateral ligament insertion at the base of the proximal phalanx. In the absence of avulsion, plain films are usually normal; degenerative changes may be present years after the injury. Referral to an orthopedist or hand surgeon is indicated for patients who have a bony fragment on X-ray that is more than 1 mm displaced or involves greater than 10% of the articular surface.

Referral is also warranted for those with lesser degrees of bony displacement but evidence of complete ligament tear (greater than 30 degrees of laxity on valgus testing or laxity greater than 15 to 20 degrees greater than the opposite thumb). The nonsurgical treatment of choice is immobilization with taping or a thumb spica splint. Immobilization should continue for two to three weeks when the patient is not performing exercises until swelling and pain have completely subsided. Once the splint is discontinued, patients should be advised to avoid heavy gripping or grasping until grip strength has returned to normal. Exposure to vibration should also be avoided.

- *Rosen's Emergency Medicine - Concepts and Clinical Practice. 8th edition. 2013. Chapter 50: Hand. 556.*

#30

You are seeing a patient with what appears to be a posterior hip dislocation. Which of the following statements is FALSE about this condition?

A. The extremity is usually abducted and externally rotated.

B. Posterior dislocations constitute 80-90% of hip dislocations.

C. Stabilization of the pelvis by an assistant greatly improves the ease of reduction.

D. Traction should be applied inferior to the knee in line with the deformity.

E. Orthopedic consultation should be obtained for hip dislocation in the presence of a fracture.

#30

Answer: A

In posterior hip dislocations, the femoral head is forced out of the acetabulum and rests posteriorly. Thus, the extremity is shortened, adducted, and internally rotated. In anterior dislocations, the extremity is abducted and externally rotated. Posterior hip dislocations constitute 80-90% of hip dislocations. When reducing the posterior dislocation with the Allis maneuver, the patient is placed supine. Downward stabilization of the pelvis is performed by an assistant, and with the knee flexed. In-line traction with gentle flexion of the hip to 90 degrees should be applied inferior to the knee. Orthopedic consultation should be obtained for hip dislocation in the presence of a fracture and with prosthetic hip dislocations, since there is a risk of loosening components of the prosthesis, fracture to the surrounding bone, and movement of the acetabular capsule.

- *Roberts and Hedges' Clinical Procedures in Emergency Medicine. 6th edition. 2013. Chapter 49: Management of Common Dislocations. 985-989.*

#31

You are seeing a patient with a lateral ankle dislocation. Which of the following statements is TRUE about this entity?

(Choose three answers.)

A. The lateral dislocation is the least common ankle dislocation seen in the ED.

B. It is the result of a significant axially loading force.

C. It is frequently associated with a malleolar fracture or a distal fibula fracture.

D. It presents with the foot laterally displaced with the skin very taut over the medial aspect of the ankle joint.

E. It is less commonly associated with rupture of the deltoid ligament.

#31
Answer: C, D, and E

Lateral ankle dislocations are the most common ankle dislocation seen in the ED, and they are usually the result of marked eversion of the foot. They are often associated with malleolar fractures or distal fibula fractures, and they are less commonly associated with rupture of the deltoid ligament. They present with the foot laterally displaced with the skin very taut over the medial aspect of the ankle joint.

To reduce this lateral dislocation:

1. Place one hand on the heel and the other on the forefoot
2. Apply longitudinal traction to the foot
3. While you have an assistant applies counter-traction to the leg, gently manipulate the foot medially; this usually produces a palpable thud to signify reduction.
4. Reassessment of neurovascular status after reduction

- *Roberts and Hedges' Clinical Procedures in Emergency Medicine. 6th edition. 2013. Chapter 49: Management of Common Dislocations. 994-995.*

#32

You are evaluating a person in whom you suspect may have a calcaneus fracture. Regarding this entity, which of the following is FALSE?

    A. If there is a fracture, Bohler's angle is usually greater than 50 degrees.

    B. If there is a fracture, Bohler's angle is likely to be less than the normal range (20-40 degrees).

    C. Calcaneal fractures are the most common tarsal fractures.

    D. Patients must be examined for concomitant injuries (e.g., spine fractures).

    E. Radiographic studies should include an AP view, a lateral view (which would show Bohler's angle), and a dedicated calcaneal view (also known as the Harris view).

#32

Answer: A

The calcaneus has 2 primary articulations, the talus and cuboid. The posterior aspect of the calcaneus is called the tuberosity. Distally, the calcaneus articulates with the cuboid. There is also a groove laterally under which the peroneus longus tendon passes. Superiorly there are 3 weight bearing facets, forming the articulation with the talus: the anterior, middle and posterior.

Bohler's angle is the complement of the angle at the apex of the posterior facet. Bohler's angle is the angle formed between two lines with the first line drawn from the superior aspect of the anterior process to the superior aspect of the posterior facet. A second line is drawn from the superior aspect of the posterior facet to the superior most point of the calcaneal tuberosity. A normal Bohler's angle is approximately 25 to 40 degrees. The angle decreases as the height of the calcaneus is lost.

Calcaneal fractures are the most common tarsal fractures. Radiographic studies should include an AP view, a lateral view (and a dedicated calcaneal view. The Harris view is obtained with the ankle in dorsiflexion and a facet posteriorly along the course of the Achilles tendon.

Although X-rays are useful, CT scanning can characterize the fractures best. Compression fractures of the spine and fractures of the proximal femur are also associated with calcaneal fractures due to axial loading force.

- Chen MY, Bohrer SP, Kelley TF. Boehler's angle: a reappraisal. Ann Emerg Med. 1991 Feb; 20(2): 122-4.

#33

Of the three types of shoulder dislocations which has the highest rate of vascular injury?

    A. Anterior

    B. Posterior

    C. Inferior

#33

Answer: C

Rare, but serious, inferior dislocations (luxatio erecta) may be due to axial force applied to an arm raised overhead. Inferior (luxatio erecta) shoulder dislocations account for only 0.5% of ED dislocations. More commonly, the shoulder is dislocated inferiorly by indirect forces abducting the arm. The neck of the humerus is levered against the acromion and the inferior capsule tears as the humeral head is forced out inferiorly.

Luxatio erecta almost always has an associated fracture or soft-tissue injury. One series found 80% of patients to have fracture of the greater tuberosity or tear of the rotator cuff. Neurologic compromise was found in 60% of patients, with the axillary nerve being most commonly injured. Inferior dislocations have the highest incidence (3.3%) of vascular compromise (axillary artery). When a brachial plexus injury is found with an inferior shoulder dislocation, there should be a high suspicion for an accompanying axillary artery injury.

- *Begaz T, Mycyk MB. Luxatio erecta: inferior humeral dislocation. J Emerg Med. 2006; 31(3): 303-4.*

- *Beeson MS. Complications of shoulder dislocation. Am J Emerg Med. 1999 May; 17(3): 288-95. full text*

Amy Kaji

#34

You are seeing a patient who you suspect may have an
Achilles tendon rupture, but when you have him walk he
still has minimal plantar flexion. Does this indicate that
he does not have an Achilles tendon rupture?

    A. Yes

    B. No

#34

Answer: B

The diagnosis of an Achilles tendon rupture is primarily clinical. Patients usually recall a sudden pain along the posterior aspect of the ankle and even hear a loud "pop". Although the pain may improve, there should be residual plantar flexion weakness. On examination, a visible and palpable tendon defect may be noted 2 to 6 cm proximal to the calcaneal insertion. Even in complete Achilles tendon rupture, patients may still have some plantar flexion strength. This is due to other intact muscles such as tibialis posterior, toe flexors, and peroneal muscles. Due to the poly-muscular strength of plantar flexion, partial tears can easily be missed.

- *Rosen's Emergency Medicine - Concepts and Clinical Practice. 8th edition. 2013. Chapter 58: Ankle and Foot. 733.*

#35

True statements about scaphoid fractures include all of the following EXCEPT:

A. There is a higher incidence of avascular necrosis and fracture nonunion in the more proximal fractures.

B. Treatment of uncomplicated, non-displaced scaphoid fractures involves immobilization in a short arm thumb spica cast.

C. Radiographic diagnosis can be difficult and a special scaphoid view should be requested when a fracture is suspected on clinical findings.

D. Scaphoid fractures are common in children.

E. Classically, physical examination reveals tenderness on palpation of the scaphoid and swelling within the anatomic snuffbox.

#35

Answer: D

Scaphoid fractures are rare in skeletally immature patients. Until late childhood and adolescence the carpal bones remain mainly cartilaginous. Physical exam may also elicit pain with palpation of the scaphoid tubercle. The major concern for scaphoid injuries is related to the risk of avascular necrosis and fracture nonunion. The blood flow to the scaphoid follows a distal to proximal pattern through the scaphoid tuberosity. More proximal and largely displaced fractures are at higher risk for avascular necrosis.

- *Rosen's Emergency Medicine - Concepts and Clinical Practice. 8th edition. 2013. Chapter 51: Wrist and Forearm. 566-567.*

#36

Regarding orthopedic illnesses in patients with HIV, which of the following statements are TRUE?

(Choose two answers.)

A. Kaposi's commonly affects the bone.

B. The most common site of musculoskeletal tuberculosis is the wrist joint.

C. HIV is thought to be an independent risk factor for reduced bone mineral density.

D. Osteonecrosis is 45 times greater in patients infected with HIV.

E. In most cases of TB osteomyelitis in HIV patients, fever is the predominant symptom.

#36

Answer: C and D

Although Kaposi's Sarcoma (KS) is the most common AIDS-associated malignancy in the US, there are only rare reports of KS involvement of the bone. Osseous KS is thought to be due to spread from other affected tissues.

In HIV, the etiology of osteopenia is multifactorial. Protease inhibitors have been linked to the development of osteopenia and osteoporosis, but HIV is thought to be an independent risk factor for reduced bone mineral density. The incidence of osteonecrosis is 45 times greater in HIV patients. Traditional risk factors include hypertriglyceridemia, corticosteroid use, and ethanol abuse. Antiretrovirals, especially protease inhibitors, have also been implicated, and osteonecrosis most often occurs in the femoral head. Osteomyelitis in the patient infected with HIV is similar to that in patients without HIV. Many organisms have been shown to cause osteomyelitis in HIV, including salmonella, cryptococcus, nocardia, candida, and tuberculosis (usually the vertebral column). In most cases of tuberculosis spinal osteomyelitis, patients are afebrile and present with isolated back pain, further complicating the diagnostic workup.

- *Takhar SS, Hendey GW. Orthopedic illnesses in patients with HIV. Emerg Med Clin N Am. 2010 May;28(2): 335-42.*

#37

Regarding orthopedic illnesses in patients with HIV, which of the following statements are TRUE?

   A. The most common organism that causes septic arthritis in HIV patients is tuberculosis.

   B. HIV patients have a higher incidence of spondyloarthropathy, which includes HLA B27 associated reactive arthritis and psoriatic arthritis.

   C. HIV-associated arthritis is a monoarticular, highly erosive arthritis that primarily affects the shoulder joints.

   D. All of the above

#37

Answer: B

The most common organism in septic arthritis is staphylococcus aureus regardless of HIV status. TB is only a common cause of septic arthritis in developing countries. HIV patients do have a higher incidence of spondyloarthropathy, including HLA B27 associated reactive arthritis (100 to 200 times more common in HIV) and psoriatic arthritis (40 times more common in HIV). HIV associated arthritis is typically a transient, self-limited nonerosive, oligoarthritis that affects the lower extremities, lasting less than 6 weeks.

- *Takhar SS, Hendey GW. Orthopedic illnesses in patients with HIV. Emerg Med Clin N Am. 2010; 28: 335-342.*

Amy Kaji

#38

Regarding orthopedic illnesses in patients with HIV, which of the following statements are TRUE?

(Choose two answers.)

    A. Polymyositis may be the first sign of HIV infection.

    B. Pyomyositis is known complication in HIV patients.

    C. The primary organism causing pyomyositis in HIV patients is streptococcus.

    D. Zidovudine-induced myopathy has distinct clinical features and is thus easy to distinguish from polymyositis.

    E. All of the above

#38
Answer: A and B

Polymyositis can occur at any stage of HIV, but it may be the first sign of HIV infection. It is an idiopathic inflammatory process of the skeletal muscle and causes a subacute progressive proximal muscle weakness with an increased creatine kinase level. Medications such as high dose zidovudine are associated with myopathies which are often clinically indistinguishable from polymyositis.

Staph aureus is the culprit organism in 90% of cases of infectious pyomyositis.

- *Takhar SS, Hendey GW. Orthopedic illnesses in patients with HIV. Emerg Med Clin N Am. 2010; 28: 335-342.*

#39

True or False: According to a study conducted at 2 academic EDs in northern California, MRSA is a common cause of septic arthritis and one distinguishing feature is the high synovial leukocyte counts.

A. True

B. False

#39

Answer: B

The median synovial fluid leukocyte count was only 15,000 in this study. The count was less than 25,000/µL in 80% of cases and it was generally much lower than in non-MRSA cases. Thus, their data suggested that treatment for MRSA be considered even when the synovial fluid leukocyte count is less than 25,000/µL.

- *Frazee BW, et al. How common is MRSA in adult septic arthritis? Ann Emerg Med. 2009; 54: 695-700. full text*

#40

According to the same study conducted at 2 academic EDs in northern California, the most common cause of septic arthritis was:

A. MRSA

B. MSSA

C. Streptococcus pneumonia

D. Enterococcus faecalis

E. Pseudomonas

#40
Answer: A

According to a cross-sectional retrospective review in 2 urban academic EDs in northern California of patients who underwent arthrocentesis in the ED from April 2006 through July 2007, when synovial fluid cultures were analyzed, MRSA was the most common organism. More specifically, 109 synovial fluid cultures were sent from the EDs. Twenty-three results (21%; 95% confidence interval [CI] 14% to 30%) were positive, of which 9 were likely contaminants; 1 was from a soft tissue abscess and 1 was from bursitis. Of 12 septic arthritis cases, 6 cultures (50%; 95% CI 21% to 78%) grew MRSA, 4 (33%; 95% CI 7% to 60%) methicillin-susceptible S aureus, and 1 each (8%; 95% CI 0% to 24%) Streptococcus pneumoniae, Enterococcus faecalis, and Pseudomonas aeruginosa. Of the 6 MRSA cases, 4 were in male patients; median age of patients was 47.5 years, 3 patients had previously diseased joints, 2 patients injected drugs, 2 patients were febrile, 3 patients had previously diseased joints, median synovial fluid leukocyte count was 15,184 cells/microL (range 3,400 to 34,075 cells/microL), and 5 patients received appropriate ED antibiotics. Note that synovial fluid cell counts were unexpectedly low in MRSA septic arthritis cases.

- Frazee BW, et al. How common is MRSA in adult septic arthritis? Ann Emerg Med. 2009 Nov; 54(5):695-700. full text

#41
A 13 year old male is seen with severe hip pain after he kicked a football (though he scored and won the game for the team). An X-ray demonstrates an isolated avulsion fracture of the lesser trochanter. TRUE statements about this entity include which of the following?

A. Most cases of this fracture occur in patients older than age 50.

B. Most cases require operative fixation.

C. Most patients present with pain in the outer thigh.

D. None of the above

#41
Answer: D

Isolated fracture of the lesser trochanter occurs when a forceful contraction of the iliopsoas muscle avulses the lesser trochanter from the physis during sudden hip flexion. 85% of all cases occur in patients younger than 20 years, with a peak incidence between the ages of 12 and 16 years. Marked tenderness can be elicited in the femoral triangle, and hip flexion against resistance is painful. Treatment of an isolated lesser trochanter avulsion fracture is usually non operative.

- *Rosen's Emergency Medicine - Concepts and Clinical Practice. 8th edition. 2013. Chapter 56: Femur and Hip. 696-697.*

#42

Hip dislocation is a true orthopedic emergency. Which of the following statements is FALSE?

A. Likelihood of avascular necrosis (AVN) is related to the degree of trauma.

B. Likelihood of AVN is related to the amount of time the femoral head remains out of joint.

C. Reduction of the hip within 6-12 hours after dislocation decreases the incidence of AVN.

D. A contraindication to hip reduction is a contralateral hip dislocation.

#42

Answer: D

The only true contraindication to hip reduction is the presence of an ipsilateral femoral neck fracture. The other three statements are true.

- *Rosen's Emergency Medicine - Concepts and Clinical Practice. 8th edition. 2013. Chapter 56: Femur and Hip. 678-691.*

#43

A 23 yo male presents with a GSW to his femur and he has an obvious deformity with > 10 cm of exposed bone and decreased pulses distally. Which of the following is appropriate management?

A. Irrigation and then coverage with saline-moistened gauze

B. Orthopedics consult

C. Update patient's tetanus status

D. Aminoglycoside in addition to first generation cephalosporin

E. All of the above

#43

Answer: E

Open fractures are divided into 3 categories: types I-III. This is a type III fracture, which is characterized by a wound > 10cm with extensive muscle devitalization and nerve and arterial involvement. The mechanism of injury is usually due to a high-energy shotgun blast or a high-velocity gunshot wound. All open wounds should be irrigated and then covered with sterile saline-moistened gauze. For all type I open fractures, a first generation cephalosporin should be administered intravenously. For type II and III fractures the recommendation is for additional gram-negative coverage due to increased tissue damage. Usually, an aminoglycoside, such as gentamicin or tobramycin, is added.

Open Fracture Types

. **Type I** - < 1 cm wound with minimal tissue damage and due to bone piercing skin

. **Type II** - 1-10 cm wound with moderate tissue damage and no arterial or nerve damage.

. **Type III** - >10cm wound with significant tissue damage with frequent nerve and arterial damage and often due to high energy blasts from gunfire.

. *Rosen's Emergency Medicine - Concepts and Clinical Practice. 8th edition. 2013. Chapter 56: Femur and Hip. 679-681.*

#44

Regarding patellar dislocations, which of the following statements is FALSE?

A. Most cases of patellar dislocations are medial dislocations, and the mechanism of injury is usually a direct blow to the anterior or medial surface of the patella.

B. Closed reduction should be attempted by directing pressure anteromedially on the lateral patellar margin, while simultaneously attempting gentle extension of the knee.

C. Hemarthrosis may be seen, particularly if there is an associated osteochondral fracture.

D. After successful reduction, the knee should be immobilized in full extension for 3-6 weeks to allow adequate time for the medial retinaculum to heal.

#44

Answer: A

Traumatic patellar dislocation is relatively common and can result from a direct blow to a flexed knee or with valgus force during external rotation. Lateral dislocations are the most common. Often the diagnosis is clinical with the knee held in flexion and the patella palpable laterally. Post reduction radiographs are useful for assessing associated fractures, specifically osteochondral fractures. After mobilization, orthopedic followup is necessary for assessment of joint laxity and instability. Adolescents are more likely to dislocate compared to the elderly.

- *Rosen's Emergency Medicine - Concepts and Clinical Practice. 8th edition. 2013. Chapter 57: Knee and Lower Leg. 699-712.*

#45

Regarding acromioclavicular (AC) joint injuries, which of the following statements is FALSE?

A. The most common mechanism of injury involves a fall or direct blow to the point of the shoulder with the arm adducted.

B. Type 1 injuries are sprains of the AC ligaments, whereas type 2 injuries disrupt the AC ligaments while the coracoclavicular (CC) ligaments remain intact.

C. Type 3 injuries involve complete disruption of the AC and CC attachments.

D. In type 4, 5, and 6 injuries, all of the ligaments and muscle attachments are disrupted.

E. Type 2 injuries warrant immediate orthopedic consult in the ED.

#45

Answer: E

Type 1, 2, and 3 injuries should be immobilized in a sling for comfort to decrease the risk of further injuries. Most patients should follow with their primary care physician and begin strength training exercises to ensure full return of range of motion. Most studies show that conservative management of type 3 injuries provides equal or in some cases, better functional results than surgical intervention.

Type 4, 5, and 6 injuries are more amenable to surgical treatment and benefit from orthopedic or sports medicine referral. In type 4 injuries, the clavicle is displaced posteriorly, superiorly in type 5 injuries, and inferiorly in type 6 injuries.

- *Rosen's Emergency Medicine - Concepts and Clinical Practice. 8th edition. 2013. Chapter 53: Shoulder 629-631.*

#46

You are seeing a patient who complains of a non-dominant left index finger injury. He states that he was using a hammer, and he accidentally hit the tip of his left index finger and nail bed. On examination, there is a > 50% subungual hematoma without any associated disruption of the nail or surrounding nail folds. The nailbed is the only area where the patient is tender, and his digital nerves appear to be intact, and the capillary refill is normal. The X-rays are negative for a fracture. The best management approach is to:

A. Prescribe antibiotics.

B. Refer to orthopedic surgery.

C. Provide pain medications and have them follow up at the community health clinic.

D. Perform a trephination.

E. Remove the nail, and place an aluminum foil or gauze impregnated with petrolatum to separate the nailfold from the nailbed.

#46

Answer: D

In the past, if the hematoma involved greater than 50% of the nail bed, the recommendations were for complete removal of the nail to ensure and repair of the under-lying laceration. However, in a study by Seaberg et al, simple nail trephination resulted in healing without any deformities or other complications in 45 patients. Now, simple nail trephination with the use of a handheld portable cautery is recommended for most subungual hematomas. A prospective study of 52 patients with nailbed injuries reported by Roser and Gellman, dem-onstrated that the outcomes were similar with nail re-moval and nail trephination, and there were significant cost savings associated with the more conservative care. Nail removal should therefore probably be reserved for subungual hematomas that are associated with disrup-tion of the nail or surrounding nailfolds.

- *Singer AJ, et al. Current management of acute cutaneous wounds. N Engl J Med. 2008 Sep 4; 359(10): 1037-46. full text*

- *Roser SE, Gellman H.Comparison of nail bed repair versus nail treph-ination for subungual hematomas in children. J Hand Surg Am. 1999 Nov; 24(6): 1166-70.*

#47

You are testing a patient's sensation for radicular symptoms. Match the following letters to the correct location to test for sensation for each nerve root.

A. L3

B. L4

C. L5

D. S1

1. Between 1st and 2nd toe

2. Lateral foot

3. Medial thigh

4. Medial foot

#47
Answer: A-3, B-4, C-1, D-2

- *Rosen's Emergency Medicine - Concepts and Clinical Practice. 8th edition. 2013. Chapter 35: Back Pain. 278-281.*

#48

You have just diagnosed a 35 yo female bungee jumper with a pilon fracture. TRUE statements about this fracture include:

(Choose four answers.)

A. One-fourth of pilon fractures are open.

B. These injuries are often comminuted with leg shortening.

C. Orthopedic consultation in the ED is necessary.

D. Early complications of pilon fractures (and post-repairs) include wound infection, skin sloughing, and pin site infection.

E. Involves the distal femoral metaphysis and usually results from a high-energy mechanism.

#48

Answer: A, B, C, and D

Pilon fractures involve the distal tibial metaphysis and are caused by a high energy mechanism. The injuries are usually comminuted and frequently are open fractures. Associated injuries include fractures of the calcaneus, tibial plateau, femoral neck, acetabulum, or lumbar vertebrae and necessitate a comprehensive trauma evaluation. The injuries are surgically repaired and require orthopedic consultation.

- *Rosen's Emergency Medicine - Concepts and Clinical Practice. 8th edition. 2013. Chapter 58: Ankle and Foot. 727-731.*

#49

You are seeing a patient who has severe leg pain that is out of proportion to that expected for the injury. Physical examination reveals tense swelling and sensory deficits. Passive dorsiflexion of the toes is painful. TRUE statements about compartment syndrome include which of the following?

A. Presence of an open wound guarantees that all compartments are decompressed.

B. The way to reliably diagnose compartment syndrome is to measure intracompartmental pressure.

C. A pressure greater than 15 mm Hg is considered diagnostic.

D. An X-ray without evidence of soft tissue swelling excludes the disease.

E. All of the above

#49

Answer: B

Patients with open wounds are still at risk for developing a compartment syndrome. A compartment that does not communicate with the wound can still develop elevated pressure. A pressure > 35 mm Hg or within 35 mm Hg of diastolic blood pressure is generally considered diagnostic. If a patient is hypotensive then compartment syndrome can occur at lower pressures and should be based on a patient's clinical picture and physical exam.

- *Rosen's Emergency Medicine - Concepts and Clinical Practice. 8th edition. 2013. Chapter 49: General Principles of Orthopedic Injuries. 521-523.*

#50

A 25 yo female fell down 8 steps and complains of foot pain. Her X-rays demonstrate sesamoid fractures of her foot under her first metatarsal. How should this be treated?

    A. Ace-wrap

    B. Weight-bearing as tolerated

    C. Hard sole shoe

    D. Below-knee walking cast

#50

Answer: D

The sesamoids are two flat oval bones located under the first metatarsal head and held within the tendon of the flexor hallucis brevis. Sesamoid fractures are uncommon and are usually caused by direct trauma or from hyperextension of the great toe. No operative interventions are needed and the fractures heal well with a short-leg walking cast.

- *Rosen's Emergency Medicine - Concepts and Clinical Practice. 8th edition. 2013. Chapter 58: Ankle and Foot. 747.*

#51

You are seeing an 80 year-old right hand dominant female who sustained a right Colles' fracture (transverse fracture of the distal radial metaphysis, which is dorsally displaced and angulated). You are not sure if the fracture needs to be reduced or not. Which of the following are criteria for reduction?

A. Intra-articular step-off > 1mm

B. Radial inclination < 15 degrees

C. Volar tilt less than neutral (0 degrees)

D. Shortening or loss of radial length greater than 2mm as compared with opposite side

E. All of the above

#51

Answer: E

In general displaced Colles' fractures requires early reduction to restore normal angulation to a neutral position. The reduction can usually be performed under conscious sedation with closed reduction. The major complication from the injury and the reduction is median nerve injury. Neurovascular function should be tested before and after reduction and orthopedics consulted if there is neurovascular injury, an open fracture, or failure to fully reduce.

- *Rosen's Emergency Medicine - Concepts and Clinical Practice. 8th edition. 2013. Chapter 51: Wrist and Forearm. 582-584.*

#52

You are seeing a 70 year old male who has a dislocated prosthetic hip. Which of the following could be associated complications?

(Choose two answers.)

A. Avascular necrosis of the femoral head

B. Traction on the sciatic nerve

C. Movement of the acetabular cup and fracturing of the surrounding bone

D. All of the above

#52

Answer: B and C

Reduction of the prosthesis hip dislocation does not generally need to happen emergently since there is replacement of the femoral head and minimal risk for avascular necrosis. However, there can be injury to the sciatic nerve. During the reduction, if attempted emergently, there can be loosening of the prosthetic components, fracture to surrounding bone, or movement of the acetabular cup. The reduction is often more difficult due to the prosthesis and is better performed in the operating room under general anesthesia.

- *Rosen's Emergency Medicine - Concepts and Clinical Practice. 8th edition. 2013. Chapter 56: Femur and Hip. 690-691.*

#53

A 26 year old man comes in complaining of midfoot pain after being tackled while playing football. He has difficulty bearing weight. Radiographs of his foot show a slight step-off at the base of the second metatarsal and middle cuneiform. Which is following is NOT true of the suspected injury described here?

A. It is likely a Lisfranc injury.

B. It occurs via either rotational forces, axial loads or crush injuries.

C. Most occur from motor vehicle crashes. Sports involving fixation of the forefoot (equestrian, windsurfing) are also associated with this type of injury.

D. Comparison X-ray views as well as weight bearing views can be help in making the diagnosis.

E. These injuries can be treated conservatively with walking boot and crutches for assistance with ambulation.

#53

Answer: E

The Lisfranc joint is made up of the articulations of the bases of the first three metatarsals with their respective cuneiforms and the 4th and 5th metatarsal with the cuboid. Intrinsic stability is provided by the associated ligaments with the second metatarsal being essential for the stability of the entire complex. Standard radiographs are usually sufficient to diagnose Lisfranc injuries.

Findings suggestive of a Lisfranc injury include widening between the first and second or second and third metatarsal or any fracture around the Lisfranc joint. Fracture of the 2nd metatarsal base is pathognomonic of occult tarsometatarsal joint disruption. This injury requires orthopedic evaluation and is usually treated with closed reduction and external fixation with non weight bearing for 3 months and an orthotic for 1 year. There is a high incidence of complications with Lisfranc injuries.

- *Rosen's Emergency Medicine - Concepts and Clinical Practice. 8th edition. 2013. Chapter 58: Ankle and Foot. 741-744.*

PEDIATRICS

#1

Regarding supraventricular tachycardia in children, which of the following statements is FALSE?

A. It is the most common symptomatic dysrhythmia in infants and children.

B. In children less than 12 years of age, the most common cause is due to Wolff-Parkinson White (WPW) syndrome.

C. The QRS complex is narrow (<0.08sec) in up to 90% of the cases.

D. No cardiac abnormalities are found in approximately half of cases.

E. The type of supraventricular tachycardia that occurs most commonly in children involves a reentrant mechanism that utilizes an accessory pathway and the atrioventricular node.

#1

Answer: B

In children less than 12 years of age, the most common cause of supraventricular tachycardia is a re-entry arrhythmia due to an accessory atrioventricular pathway, causing SVT. No cardiac abnormalities are found in 50% of patients, and WPW is present in only 10-20% of cases.

· *Rosen's Emergency Medicine - Concepts and Clinical Practice. 8th edition. 2013. Chapter 171: Cardiac Disorders. 2155.*

#2

Regarding pediatric head trauma patients, which of the following were predictors of "very low risk for clinically significant injury in children less than 2 years of age"?

A. Normal mental status

B. No scalp hematoma except frontal

C. No loss of consciousness or loss of consciousness < 5 seconds

D. Non-severe injury mechanism

E. No palpable skull fracture

F. All of the above

#2

Answer: F

In addition, the child should be acting normally according to the parents. If all were present, the negative predictive value was 100% (95%CI 99.7-100%).

The prediction rule for children aged 2 years and older included:

1. Normal mental status
2. No loss of consciousness
3. No vomiting
4. Non-severe injury mechanism
5. No signs of basilar skull fracture
6. No severe headache.

This rule for those greater than 2 years of age had a negative predictive value of 99.95% (95% CI 99.81-99.99%). Neither rule (for <2yo or >2yo) missed neurosurgical interventions in the validation cohort.

• *Kuppermann N, et al. Identification of children at very low risk of clinically-important brain injuries after head trauma: a prospective cohort study. Lancet. 2009; 374(9696): 1160-1170. full text*

• *WikEM - PECARN Head CT Rule http://wikem.org/wiki/ EBQ:PECARN_Pediatric_Head_CT_Rule*

#3

The most common cause of symptomatic bradycardia in infants and children is:

A. Hypothermia

B. Congenital heart blocks

C. Medications

D. Hypoxia

E. Toxins

#3

Answer: D

In pediatrics, hypoxia is the most common cause of bradycardia. Thus, ensuring adequate oxygenation and ventilation is paramount. This should be performed before any attempts at external pacing. In children, epinephrine is the first line medication, if the patient is not responsive to respiratory support. Children also have a greater risk of hypothermia, and adequate warming should be provided. Other causes of bradycardia include, increased intracranial pressure, heart blocks, and medication and toxin ingestion.

- *Rosen's Emergency Medicine - Concepts and Clinical Practice. 8th edition. 2013. Chapter 171: Cardiac Disorders. 2155.*

#4

Regarding intussusception, which of the following is FALSE?

A. The triad of paroxysmal abdominal pain, vomiting, and rectal bleeding is found in over 90% of patients.

B. Early diagnosis is essential, since the duration of intussusception affects morbidity and mortality.

C. A negative guaiac does not exclude the diagnosis but a positive stool guaiac increases the likelihood of intussusception.

D. Air and barium enema reductions have success rates from 65% to 90%.

E. A normal plain abdominal radiograph does not exclude intussusception.

#4

Answer: A

The classic triad of intussusception of paroxysmal abdominal pain, vomiting, and rectal bleeding is present in less than a third patients. Only 85% manifest paroxysmal abdominal pain, and only 75% experience vomiting. Rectal bleeding is an even less constant feature and may only be seen in 40% of patients.

• *Harwood-Nuss' Clinical Practice of Emergency Medicine 5th edition. 2010. Chapter 259: Intussusception. 1265-1266.*

#5

Which of the following is NOT a risk factor for cerebral edema in diabetic ketoacidosis (DKA)?

A. Elevated blood urea nitrogen

B. Low serum potassium on presentation

C. Treatment with bicarbonate

D. Age < 3 years

E. Failure of serum sodium to rise steadily with correction of hyperglycemia

#5

Answer: B

Patients in DKA may present with hypo-, eu-, or hyper-kalemia. Cerebral edema is the most serious immediate risk to the child in DKA, occurring in 1% of cases. The presentation can include altered mental status, focal neurologic deficits, and abnormal respiratory pattern. The mortality of cerebral edema is 25%, and of those who survive, 25% will have significant morbidity. Treatment includes airway management and mannitol 1 g/kg IV given over 10 minutes. Patients should be admitted to an intensive care unit.

Despite multiple investigations and changes in the therapy of DKA, the incidence of cerebral edema has not changed in the past two decades. Risk factors for cerebral edema in DKA are:

- Elevated BUN

- Low pCO_2

- Treatment with bicarbonate

- Failure of measured serum sodium to rise steadily with correction of hyperglycemia

- Age < 3 years

- New-onset diabetes

- *Marcin JP, et al. Factors associated with adverse outcomes in children with diabetic ketoacidosis-related cerebral edema. Journal of Pediatrics. 2002; 141(6): 793-797.*

#6

You are seeing a 5 year old child who is brought in by his parents for petechiae and easy bruising. There is no fever, night sweats, headache, or any weight loss. On examination, he is well-appearing, afebrile, and has scattered petechiae over his chest and ecchymosis on his legs. The CBC is notable for a platelet count of $10\times10^3/mm^3$. You suspect acute immune thrombocytopenia purpura (ITP). The least appropriate diagnostic and management step is to:

A. Administer steroids

B. Administer IVIG

C. Transfuse platelets

D. Administer anti-Rho D immune globulin

E. Obtain a Coombs test

#6

Answer: C

The only indication for platelet transfusions is the presence of life-threatening hemorrhage, such as intracranial hemorrhage. Large doses are often required because normal doses are ineffective due to platelet destruction. The presence of one or more of the following factors is used as an indication for pharmacologic intervention:

- Presence of severe or life-threatening bleeding
- Planned procedure that is likely to induce blood loss
- Concomitant bleeding dyscrasia (eg, hemophilia)

The ideal pharmacologic therapy is corticosteroids, IVIG, or intravenous intravenous anti-Rho(D) immune globulin. These interventions may shorten the duration of symptoms. Most emergency physicians are not familiar with the recommendation for Anti-Rho(D) Ig, but it has been shown to be effective in the treatment of children with ITP in high doses. However, anti-Rho(D) Ig is associated with an increased incidence of significant hemolysis and should be used in consultation with a hematologist and only in patients with a hemoglobin level greater than 10 g/dL.

The most commonly recommended dosage of IVIG is administration as a single dose of 1000 mg/kg. Inpatient work-up will include a Coombs antibody test to identify the rare patient with Evans syndrome. All patients should be admitted for further workup and monitoring for bleeding.

- Neunert C, et al. The American Society of Hematology 2011 evidence-based practice guideline for immune thrombocytopenia. Blood. 2011; 117(16): 4190-4207.

#7

The parents of the 4 year old child with the febrile seizure would like to know what the chances are of their daughter for having another febrile seizure. You state that the factors that increase her risk for recurrence are all of the following EXCEPT:

A. Young age at onset

B. History of febrile seizures in a first-degree relative

C. Low degree of fever while in the emergency department

D. Brief duration between the onset of fever and the initial seizure

E. Complex features

#7

Answer: E

Any child who has a febrile seizure is at risk for future febrile seizures. The recurrence rate is estimated at 35% overall. Children who are younger than 1 year old at first presentation may have as high as a 65% chance of a recurrence. Most recurrent febrile seizures take place within the first year of occurrence. A prospective cohort study of 428 children with a first febrile seizure determined four factors that increase the recurrence risk:

1. Young age at onset,
2. History of febrile seizures in a first-degree relative,
3. Low degree of fever while in the emergency department
4. Brief duration between the onset of fever and the initial seizure.

Children who had all four factors were much more likely to have a recurrent febrile seizure than those with none. Complex features were not associated with the risk of recurrence.

Febrile seizures are divided into two categories, simple, or complex, based upon clinical features. Simple febrile seizures must be less than 15 minutes, have no focal features, and there should only be one over a 24hr period. Complex febrile seizures are characterized by lasting more than 15 minutes, have focal features, and may recur multiple times in a 24hr period.

• Berg AT, et al. Predictors of recurrent febrile seizures. A prospective cohort study. Arch Pediatr Adolesc Med. 1997; 151(4): 371-378.

• Chung, S. Febrile Seizure. Korean J Pediatr. Sep 2014; 57(9): 384–395. full text

#8

You are seeing a 6 year old female whom you believe may have Henoch-Schönlein Purpura (HSP). Which of the following is NOT a classic symptom or lab characteristic of this vasculitic disease?

A. Thrombocytopenia

B. Palpable purpura

C. Renal disease (proteinuria, hematuria)

D. Arthralgias

E. Abdominal pain

#8

Answer: A

Henoch-Schönlein Purpura (HSP) is the most common systemic vasculitis of childhood. It is a self-limited disease and is characterized by a tetrad of clinical manifestations that vary in their occurrence and order of presentation. The disease is characterized by a tetrad of clinical manifestations:

1. Palpable purpura (without thrombocytopenia)
2. Arthritis/arthralgia
3. Abdominal pain
4. Renal disease

The abdominal pain associated with HSP is caused by submucosal hemorrhage. The common areas affected are the duodenum, stomach, colon and terminal ileum. Intussusception is the most common complication of HSP.

• Davin JC, et al. Henoch-Schönlein purpura nephritis in children. Nat Rev Nephrol. 2014; 10(10): 563-573.

#9

You are seeing a 4 week old with colicky abdominal pain with streaks of blood in the diaper. You think of intussusception. You try to remember the peak incidence of this disease and wonder if the child is in the right age range. You recall that intussusception is the most common cause of bowel obstruction in the:

    A. 2 – 8 week age group

    B. 2 month – 4 month age group

    C. 4 year old – 12 year old

    D. 6 months to 12 months

    E. 6 years - 8 years

#9

Answer: D

Intussusception is the most common cause of intestinal obstruction in infants. It occurs generally in patients less than 2 years old and most commonly between the ages of 5 months to 12 months of age. Approximately 60 % of children are younger than one year old, and 80% are younger than two.

- *Rosen's Emergency Medicine - Concepts and Clinical Practice. 8th edition. 2013. Chapter 172: Gastrointestinal Disorders. 2176-2178.*

#10

The benefits of dexamethasone treatment for moderate-to-severe croup are well established. Which of the following statements is FALSE?

A. At least 60% of children with croup who present for emergency care have mild symptoms and are routinely discharged without observation and often without treatment.

B. Corticosteroids for moderate-to-severe croup, result in reduction in the frequency and duration of hospitalization.

C. The risk of corticosteroid administration exceeds the benefit for patients with mild croup and should thus be avoided.

D. Corticosteroid treatment for lung disease in premature neonates has been associated with long-term adverse effects on growth and neuromotor and cognitive function.

E. Repeated short courses of oral corticosteroids in children with asthma are not associated with long-term negative effects on bone metabolism, bone density, or adrenal function.

#10

Answer: C

Bjornsen et al conducted a double-blind trial at four pediatric emergency departments in which 720 children with mild croup were randomly assigned to receive one oral dose of either dexamethasone (0.6 mg per kilogram of body weight) or placebo. The children had mild croup, as defined by a score of 2 on the croup scoring system of Westley, et al (defined as the presence of a barking cough, no audible stridor at rest, and mild or no indrawing of the chest wall). The primary outcome was a return to a medical care provider for croup within seven days after treatment. The secondary outcome was the presence of ongoing symptoms of croup on days 1, 2, and 3 after treatment. Other outcomes included economic costs, hours of sleep lost by the child, and stress on the part of the parent. Baseline clinical characteristics were similar in the two groups. In the dexamethasone group, there was quicker resolution of croup symptoms (P=0.003), less lost sleep (P<0.001), and less stress on the part of the parent (P<0.001).

The authors of this study concluded that dexamethasone is an effective treatment that results in consistent and small but important clinical and economic benefits. Although the long-term effects of this treatment are not known, data support the use of dexamethasone in most, if not all, children with croup.

• LLSA 2006: Bjornsen CL, et al. A randomized trial of a single dose of oral dexamethasone for mild croup. N Engl J Med. 2004 Sep 23; 351(13): 1306-13.

#11

The method of choice to diagnose intussusception in most institutions is:

A. KUB

B. Barium enema

C. CT scan

D. Ultrasound

E. UGI

#11

Answer: D

Ultrasonography is the initial diagnostic modality to detect intussusception. The sensitivity and specificity approach 100%, and ultrasound is better than fluoroscopy at detecting the lead point. The characteristic ultrasound findings are a "bull's eye" or "coiled spring," which represent layers of the intestine that have intussuscepted.

An intussusception can be seen on CT, but CT exposes the patient to unnecessary radiation and will not aid in treating the disease. Reduction of intussusception is by either fluoroscopy or ultrasound, and either contrast or air enemas may be used.

* *Rosen's Emergency Medicine - Concepts and Clinical Practice. 8th edition. 2013. Chapter 172: Gastrointestinal Disorders. 2176-2178.*

#12

You have now diagnosed your child with intussusception via ultrasound. You now decide to order a non-operative reduction using either contrast or air enema technique, depending upon which pediatric radiologist is in-house. Risk factors for non-reduction include which of the following?

A. If the patient is < 1 year of age

B. If the child is older than 5 years of age

C. If the plain films demonstrate signs of intestinal obstruction

D. Ileo-ileo-colic intussusception

E. All of the above

#12

Answer: E

Reduction is usually successful in patients with ileocolic intussusception. However, ileo-ileo-colic and jejuno-ileol intussusception reduction is often more difficult. Younger children (less than 3 months) and older children (greater than 5 years) may also be more difficult to reduce. Additionally, the presence of signs of bowel obstruction and a longer duration of symptoms (especially if >48 hrs) decreases the likelihood of successful reduction.

• *Rosen's Emergency Medicine - Concepts and Clinical Practice. 8th edition. 2013. Chapter 172: Gastrointestinal Disorders. 2176-2178.*

#13

You are seeing a 20 month old with a history of gastroschisis and resultant short gut syndrome. He has total parenteral nutrition (TPN) infusing and is being admitted for line sepsis. The troubled parents ask you what is the likelihood of the child transitioning to an oral diet. Which of the following are predictors of transitioning to an oral diet?

A. The length of remaining small bowel

B. The remaining segments of small bowel and intestinal continuity

C. Presence of the colon and an intact ileocecal valve

D. Intestinal adaptation

E. All of the above

Amy Kaji

#13

Answer: E

There are many factors that determine the successful transition to oral feedings in patient suffering from short gut syndrome. Factors include:

1. Length of small bowel
2. Presence of the colon
3. Intact ileocecal valve
4. Degree of intestinal adaptation

Overall intestinal length is the greatest determining factor. The ileum is the site for absorption of vitamin B12 and bile salts and its resection causes the greatest amount of malabsorption of fat-soluble vitamins. The colon contributes most to water and electrolyte absorption. The ileocecal valve helps regulate small intestinal transit times and further contributes to nutrient absorption.

• *Quirós-Tejeira RE, et al. Long-term parenteral nutritional support and intestinal adaptation in children with short bowel syndrome: a 25-year experience. J Pediatr. 2004 Aug; 145(2): 157-63.*

#14
Regarding bronchiolitis, which of the following statements is FALSE?

A. Risk factors associated with more severe disease include prematurity < 34 weeks, a history of cyanosis, congenital heart disease, a respiratory rate > 70, and an oxygen saturation < 95%.

B. Children with severe disease should be allowed to assume a position of comfort, and 100% oxygen should be delivered.

C. If the child presents on the first day of illness, they are unlikely to progress.

D. Less than half of infants with bronchiolitis will respond to bronchodilators.

E. Infants less than 2 months of age are at risk for apnea and admission should be strongly considered.

#14

Answer: C

It is important to identify whether the child is in the first few days of illness. If they present on day 3 to 5 day, then the illness has most likely peaked and will generally not worsen. Early on in disease, especially during the first day, children should have 24hr follow up arranged, as symptoms can certainly worsen. Unfortunately, there is no strong or convincing evidence of effectiveness for any treatment for bronchiolitis, other than supportive care.

- *Ralston S, et al. Clinical Practice Guideline: The Diagnosis, Management, and Prevention of Bronchiolitis. Pediatrics. 2014; 134(5): 1474-1502. full text*

#15

Vomiting limits the success of rehydration in children with gastroenteritis. In a randomized controlled trial of orally disintegrating tablets of ondansetron, which of the following was NOT demonstrated to be statistically significantly different between the groups?

    A. Likelihood of vomiting

    B. Frequency of vomiting

    C. Rate of hospitalization and rate of return visits to the emergency department

    D. Mean length of stay in the emergency department

    E. Treatment with intravenous hydration

#15

Answer: C

As compared with children who received placebo, children who received ondansetron were less likely to vomit (14% vs. 35%; relative risk, 0.40; 95% confidence interval, 0.26 to 0.61). The children had greater oral intake (239 ml vs. 196 ml, P=0.001) and were less likely to be treated by intravenous rehydration (14% vs. 31%; relative risk, 0.46; 95% confidence interval, 0.26 to 0.79).

The mean length of stay in the emergency department was reduced by 12% in the ondansetron group, as compared with the placebo group (P=0.02). However the rates of hospitalization (4% and 5%, respectively; P=1.00) and return visits to the emergency department (19% and 22%, P=0.73) did not differ significantly between the groups.

. LLSA 2008: Freedman SB, et al. Oral ondansetron for gastroenteritis in a pediatric emergency department. N Engl J Med. 2006; 354: 1698-1705.

#16
Indications for hospitalization for HSP include:

    A. Elevated creatinine with significant proteinuria

    B. Severe gastrointestinal bleeding

    C. Severe abdominal pain

    D. Changes in mental status

    E. All of the above.

Amy Kaji

#16

Answer: E

The main treatment of Henoch-Schönlein purpura is supportive care for pain relief and oral hydration. Patients should be hospitalized if they cannot tolerate oral hydration or if they have severe abdominal pain or renal failure. However, most patients can be cared for as outpatients. In the rare case, patients may develop gastrointestinal bleeding, altered mental status or renal insufficiency with (elevated creatinine, hypertension, or proteinuria). Oral prednisone (1 to 2 mg/kg per day) may be used for children who are refractory to supportive care.

- Rosen's Emergency Medicine - Concepts and Clinical Practice. 8th edition. 2013. Chapter 172: Gastrointestinal Disorders. 2180-2181.

#17

A 7 month old female is brought in by her mother because she is lethargic and only weakly cries to painful stimulation. Mother also noted poor feeding and that she was like a "rag doll" today. She notes the child had been given honey with her morning toast for the past two days. Which of the following is FALSE regarding your suspected case of botulism?

A. Infantile botulism results from ingestion of C. botulinum spores, which are able to germinate and produce toxin in the high pH of the GI tract of infants.

B. Botulinum toxin works by binding irreversibly to the presynaptic membrane of peripheral nerves and cranial nerves.

C. Botulism classically features an ascending, symmetric paralysis.

D. The toxin decreases cholinergic output, and anticholinergic signs such as constipation, urinary retention, dry skin, increased temperature and dilated pupils may be seen.

E. Initial treatment is focused on stabilizing the airway and initiating supportive measures.

#17

Answer: C

Botulism classically presents as a descending symmetric paralysis. In infantile botulism, the spores germinate in the GI tract due to a higher pH compared to adults. Infantile botulism occurs in children up to 11 months of age. Spores are able to survive in honey, which is why it is recommended that infants under the age of 1 years old avoid consumption. This diagnosis must be in the differential of the floppy infant. Treatment is focused on protecting the airway and supportive measures in a critical care setting. Antitoxin can shorten the course of disease.

- *Rosen's Emergency Medicine - Concepts and Clinical Practice. 8th edition. 2013. Chapter 129: Bacteria. 1704-1707.*

- *WHO Botulism Fact Sheet - http://www.who.int/mediacentre/factsheets/fs270/en/*

#18

Acute otitis media (AOM) is the most common diagnosis for which antibiotics are prescribed for children. A trial that evaluated a "wait-and-see prescription" (WASP) for antibiotics vs. standard treatment in which antibiotics were prescribed (SP) from the ED. The parents of WASP group were asked not to fill the prescription unless the child was not better in 48 hours. Which of the following results were noted?

A. Substantially more parents in the WASP group did not fill the antibiotic prescription.

B. There was no significant difference between the two groups in rates of fever, otalgia, or unscheduled visits for medical care.

C. Within the WASP group, fever and otalgia were significantly associated with filling the antibiotic prescription.

D. A, B, and C

E. None of the above

#18

Answer: D

In a study of 283 patients who were randomized either to the WASP group (n = 138) or the SP group (n = 145), more parents in the WASP group did not fill the antibiotic prescription (62% vs 13%; P<.001). There was no statistically significant difference between the groups in the frequency of subsequent fever, otalgia, or unscheduled visits for medical care. Within the WASP group, both fever (relative risk [RR], 2.95; 95% confidence interval [CI], 1.75 - 4.99; P<.001) and otalgia (RR, 1.62; 95% CI, 1.26 - 2.03; P<.001) were associated with filling the prescription. Note that all patients received ibuprofen and otic analgesic drops for use at home.

- *LLSA 2008: Spiro DM, et al. Wait and see prescription approach for acute otitis media: a randomized controlled trial. JAMA. 2006; 296: 1235-1241.*

#19

Regarding meconium aspiration, which of the following statements is FALSE?

A. The need for tracheal intubation should be made based on the consistency of the meconium (thick vs. thin).

B. Aspiration of meconium can be avoided by aggressive intervention to avoid aspiration.

C. As soon as the infant's head is delivered, the mouth and the nose should be suctioned.

D. Meconium in the amniotic fluid is a sign of in-utero distress.

E. The presence of thick or particulate meconium before or at delivery immediately should raise concern about the potential for aspiration.

#19

Answer: A

The need for endotracheal intubation with tracheal suctioning after delivery of the infant should be made based on the vigor of the infant, rather than on the consistency of the meconium. Tracheal suctioning should be performed in any neonate with meconium stained fluid and:

1. Absent or depressed respiration,
2. Poor muscle tone
3. Heart rate less than 100 beats/minute.

A meconium aspirator can be attached to an endotracheal tube and connected to wall suction at 100 mm Hg or less. The ETT is withdrawn as suction is being applied with re-intubation and suction repeated until the meconium clears. Generally two passes are enough to clear the meconium.

- *Rosen's Emergency Medicine - Concepts and Clinical Practice. 8th edition. 2013. Chapter 11: Neonatal Resuscitation. 113-114.*

#20
Regarding roseola infantum (exanthem subitum), which of the following statements is FALSE?

A. It occurs most commonly on children between 6 months and 2 years of age.

B. Parvovirus B19 is the primary etiologic agent.

C. Classic roseola has a characteristic history of high fever for 3 to 5 days, followed by defervescence that coincides with the onset of rash.

D. The rash typically consists of small, discrete, rose-pink macules or morbilliform (maculo-papular) distributed primarily on the trunk before spreading to the rest of the body.

E. Febrile seizures occur in 10-15% of cases.

Amy Kaji

#20

Answer: B

HHV-6 is the primary agent, although HHV-7 can cause a similar illness. Parvovirus B19 causes erythema infectiosum (fifth disease).

- *Harwood-Nuss' Clinical Practice of Emergency Medicine 5th edition. 2010. Chapter 271: Rashes: Maculopapular Lesions and Infestations. 1314.*

#21

You are seeing a "floppy infant": an infant with decreased tone and strength. TRUE statements about this presentation include which of the following:

A. Hypotonia and weakness can present as decreased activity, poor suck or choking, weak cry, respiratory distress, constipation, decreased head movement, or decreased eye movement.

B. Cerebral hemorrhage could be a cause

C. Infantile botulism could be a cause

D. Sepsis could be a cause

E. All of the above

#21

Answer: E

Other causes include brain malformation, spinal cord injury, spinal muscular atrophy, neonatal myasthenia, mitochondrial diseases, muscular dystrophy, Prader Willi, electrolyte disturbances, and metabolic disorders.

• *Harwood-Nuss' Clinical Practice of Emergency Medicine 5th edition. 2010. Chapter 264: Newborn Problems. 1294-1295.*

#22
Regarding apparent life-threatening events (ALTE) in children, which of the following is FALSE?

A. "Apparent life-threatening event" (ALTE) is not a specific diagnosis, but a constellation of symptoms that describe an abrupt change in an infant's breathing, color, and state.

B. ALTEs are thought to be causally related to SIDS.

C. The caregivers of infants who have had an ALTE should receive training in standard cardiopulmonary resuscitation (CPR) for infants.

D. Caregivers of infants who have had an ALTE should also be instructed in safe infant care practices, including supine sleep position with face free, safe sleeping environments and elimination of tobacco smoke exposure..

E. When an infant suffers recurrent, severe ALTE events requiring cardiopulmonary resuscitation (CPR) the diagnosis of intentional suffocation (child abuse) must be considered.

#22

Answer: B

ALTE refers to a range problems ranging from benign to near-fatal, whereas SIDS denotes a fatal problem. A specific cause for the ALTE can be identified in over half of patients after a careful history, physical examination, and appropriate laboratory evaluation. Most episodes are caused by gastroesophageal reflux, neurologic problems (such as seizures or breath-holding spells), and infection.

Although an association between SIDS and ALTE had been suggested, the majority of SIDS victims do not experience apnea prior to death. No study has be able to confirm a causal relationship between the two processes.

. *Fu LY, et al. Apparent life-threatening events: an update. Pediatr Rev. 2012 Aug; 33(8): 361-8.*

#23

Certain exanthems present classically in the pediatric population. Which of the following diseases are NOT correctly paired with their presentation?

A. **Measles (rubeola)** - associated with a blanching erythematous "brick-red" maculopapular rash beginning in the head and neck area and spreading to the trunk and extremities; patients may also have fever, cough, coryza, and conjunctivitis.

B. **Chickenpox** - characterized by classic vesicular lesions on an erythematous base that appear in crops and are present in different stages from papules through vesicles to crusting.

C. **Rubella** - rash resembles measles; prominent postauricular, posterior cervical, and/or suboccipital adenopathy.

D. **Roseola infantum or exanthem subitum** – rash due to human herpesvirus 6 or 7, primarily seen in infants, is characterized by high fever for three to four days, followed by seizures and a generalized maculopapular rash that spreads from the trunk to the extremities but spares the face.

E. None of the above

#23

Answer: E

All of the disease entities above are correctly paired with their presentations.

. *Harwood-Nuss' Clinical Practice of Emergency Medicine 5th edition. 2010. Chapter 271: Rashes: Maculopapular Lesions and Infestations. 1311-1315.*

#24

Foreign bodies swallowed in the esophagus would be expected to lodge at all of the following places EXCEPT:

A. At the upper esophageal sphincter

B. At the lower esophageal sphincter

C. At the take-off of the superior mesenteric artery

D. At the aortic arch

E. At a previously identified stricture

#24

Answer: C

Esophageal foreign bodies will lodge at narrowed areas such as the upper esophageal sphincter (cricopharyngeus muscle), the level of the aortic arch, and the lower esophageal sphincter. If an object has remain lodged in the middle third of the esophagus, it suggests an esophageal stricture. Children with food boluses stuck in the esophagus may have an underlying stricture if there were prior surgical procedures performed as an infant. Tracheoesophageal fistulas, although uncommon, are a potential anatomic cause of obstruction.

- *Rosen's Emergency Medicine - Concepts and Clinical Practice. 8th edition. 2013. Chapter 60: Foreign Bodies. 776 - 781.*

#25

Which of the following is NOT part of the classic tetrad of Henoch-Schonlein purpura (HSP)?

- A. Fever

- B. Arthralgia/arthritis

- C. Abdominal pain

- D. Renal disease

- E. Palpable purpura without thrombocytopenia

#25

Answer: A

Henoch-Schönlein purpura (HSP) is the most common systemic vasculitis of childhood. HSP is self-limited and is characterized by a tetrad of clinical manifestations that may be present at varying times during the disease course:

1. Palpable purpura
2. Arthralgia and/or arthritis
3. Abdominal pain
4. Renal disease

Management of HSP is divided into supportive care, symptomatic therapy, and targeted therapy depending on disease progression.

• Rosen's Emergency Medicine - Concepts and Clinical Practice. 8th edition. 2013. Chapter 172: Gastrointestinal Disorders. 2180-2181.

#26

A three-week-old boy full term, normal vaginal delivery and no complications at birth, is brought in by his father because he received a letter in the mail about some abnormal laboratory test results. The baby also apparently has not been eating well, has prolonged periods of "increased crying," and vomits before feedings. The physical exam is significant for a sleepy newborn with hyper-pigmentation of the skin, including the scrotum. His weight is 3.7 kg, which is lower than his birth weight. What is the most appropriate management?

A. Do a head-to-toe exam looking for causes of "increased crying", and, if negative, refer to his pediatrician.

B. Check the baby's blood glucose, and if normal and eating in the ED, refer to his pediatrician.

C. After a thorough history and physical, refer to Failure to Thrive clinic if negative.

D. Draw blood for serum chemistry, complete blood count, total bilirubin, urine test, in addition to a head-to-toe exam.

#26

Answer: D

In most states in the U.S., the newborn screening includes tests for congenital adrenal hyperplasia. However, the assays have a two- to three-week turn-around time (perhaps longer if the parents are hard to contact). In this patient with poor feeding, poor weight gain, vomiting, (and possibly inappropriate hyper-pigmentation) should suggest the diagnosis of possible missed adrenal hyperplasia.

Various enzymes are involved in the production of cortisol. If there is a congenital absence of these enzymes, there is no feedback from the adrenals to the hypothalamic-pituitary axis (HPA). Without negative feedback, ACTH is secreted by the HPA, which in turn acts on the adrenals. The result is a hyperplastic adrenal gland that is partially non-functioning and lacks the enzymes needed to convert cortisol into corticosteroids, mineralocorticoids, and sex steroids.

Baby girls can be more readily diagnosed in the nursery (before the screening labs) due to the appearance of virilization if congenital adrenal hyperplasia was present. Baby boys can be overlooked, since they may outwardly appear normal. Treatment is geared towards the clinical presentation of the child – fluid resuscitation and correction of hyperkalemia, hypoglycemia, and acidosis is often required. Hydrocortisone administration in the ED based on the presumed diagnosis is appropriate for the ill neonate. The initial bolus of hydrocortisone is 2 mg/kg IM/IV.

- Rosen's Emergency Medicine - Concepts and Clinical Practice. 8th edition. 2013. Chapter 128: Thyroid and Adrenal Disorders. 2180-2181.

#27

A 7 year-old girl took some of her mother's medications for hypothyroidism. She is febrile, has bounding pulses, widened pulse pressure, diaphoretic, restless, and screaming at the nurse putting in an IV. What is the correct order of treatment?

A. C-collar, backboard, and CT scan

B. Propranolol, iodide, dexamethasone, call Endocrine

C. Propranolol, IVF, monitor

D. Propranolol, iodide, methimazole or PTU, call Endocrine

E. Radioactive iodine treatment

#27

Answer: C

This child overdosed on exogenous thyroid hormone. Treatment is focused on addressing the autonomic signs and symptoms with propranolol and providing supportive care until she metabolizes the drug. Thyroid storm due to endogenous hyperthyroidism is uncommon in children, and so treatment largely follows adult guidelines. Propranolol treats the autonomic surge and has the additional benefit of inhibiting the peripheral conversion of T4 (most abundant form of thyroid hormone) to T3 (the most active form of thyroid hormone). Propylthiouracil works centrally at the thyroid gland to prevent further thyroid hormone synthesis, and inhibits the conversion of T4 to T3. Iodide will terminate thyroid hormone release. However, if PTU is not given at least an hour before iodide, the thyroid gland will absorb the iodide and continue to make more hormones, and potentially worsen symptoms Methimazole is an alternative agent to PTU and in adults, is now the preferred agent due to the risk of liver toxicity with PTU. For pediatrics, PTU should be avoided. Dexamethasone inhibits hormone release and conversion.

• *Rosen's Emergency Medicine - Concepts and Clinical Practice. 8th edition. 2013. Chapter 128: Thyroid and Adrenal Disorders. 1678-1684.*

#28

You are about to intubate a young child with succinyl-choline and a medical student asks you why you are going to administer atropine. You state:

    A. It is to decrease secretions.

    B. It will decrease the cough reflex.

    C. It will decrease airway hyperresponsiveness.

    D. It will potentially prevent bradycardia.

    E. None of the above

#28

Answer: D

Children are susceptible to a bradycardic response to both succinylcholine and laryngoscopic manipulation. This response occurs from increased vagal tone. To decrease the likelihood of this response, the use of a vagolytic agent, such as atropine, has been recommended when rapid sequence intubation is performed in children. The use of atropine is not based on strong evidence. The current recommendation for children under 10 years of age undergoing RSI is that atropine 0.02 mg/kg be given intravenously three minutes before intubation.

• Allen KA. Premedication for Neonatal Intubation: Which Medications are Recommended and Why? Adv Neonatal Care. 2012; 12(2): 107–111.

#29

You are seeing a 6 week old who is brought in by worried parents for inconsolable crying and fussiness for the last several hours. The baby was full term and has been feeding well, and there had been good weight gain. The parents ask you whether this could be colic. Wessel's criteria for the diagnosis of colic includes all of the following:

A. Age less than 3 months

B. Crying more than 3 hours daily for more than 3 weeks

C. Both of the above

D. Neither of the above

#29

Answer: C

All babies cry, but the amount of crying increases from 2-3 hours daily when the child is 6-8 weeks of age and then tapers off fairly soon after that. Young babies tend to cry more later in the day, in late afternoon or evening. Wessel's criteria for the diagnosis of colic includes:

1. Age less than 3 months
2. Crying more than 3 hours daily for more than 3 weeks.

Often the diagnosis is unclear in the ED but if any of the two criteria are present the patient should be searched for any potential metabolic causes, signs of abuse, cardiac dysrhythmias, corneal abrasions, hernias, torsion, acute abdominal process, hair tourniquets, or malnutrition.

- *Roberts DM, et al. Infantile Colic. Am Fam physician. 2004; 70(4): 735-740. full text*

#30

Congenital heart disease can be categorized into cyanotic and acyanotic. Which of the following are categorized as cyanotic?

(Choose two answers.)

    A. Truncus arteriosus

    B. ASD

    C. VSD

    D. Coarctation of the aorta

    E. Tetralogy of Fallot

#30

Answer: A and E

Tetralogy of Fallot and Truncus Arteriosus are cyanotic. Tetralogy is the most common form of cyanotic CHD, and the abnormalities associated with it are a large VSD, right ventricular outflow obstruction, right ventricular hypertrophy and an overriding aorta. Truncus arteriosus is one of two main mixing lesions (the other one is total anomalous pulmonary venous return (TAPVR)). Significant mixing of desaturated blood with the systemic-bound blood causes the cyanosis, and they are accompanied by an obstruction to pulmonary blood flow and therefore, suboptimal oxygenation of the blood, which compounds the cyanosis. Both TA and TAPVR are not ductal-dependent lesions, and therefore, they do not respond to PGE1. TA and TAPVR constitute less than 2% of all CHD.

ASD and VSD are left-to-right shunt lesions (other examples are PDA and endocardial cushion defects). Any defect in the interventricular septum, whether at the atrial or ventricular level will cause an acyanotic shunt, with blood flowing from the left to the right heart. The volume of blood that is shunted will determine the degree of chamber enlargement and hypertrophy. The greater the flow, the more likely you will hear a murmur. The amount of flow also dictates the timing and manner of presentation. Higher flows will cause earlier and more severe CHF presentations.

- *Rosen's Emergency Medicine - Concepts and Clinical Practice. 8th edition. 2013. Chapter 171: Cardiac Disorders. 2146-2151.*

#31

You are evaluating an infant with cyanosis. On presentation, the room air oxygen saturation of the infant was less than 85% and there was no increase in pulse oximetry with 10 minutes of administration of 100% oxygen. You then decide to begin treatment with PGE1. After you begin treatment the infant becomes apneic. You should then:

A. Decreased the dose of infusion, as apnea is dose-related.

B. Intubate the patient.

#31

Answer: B

Apnea is a common side effect of PGE1 and occurs in 12%. PGE-1 associated apnea is not dose related. Thus, if the patient develops apnea, instead of decreasing an effective dose, the patient should be intubated. Apnea usually occurs within the first few hours of PGE1 treatment but can occur at any time during its administration. PGE1 can also cause hypotension, bradycardia, hyperpyrexia, and flushing.

- *Rosen's Emergency Medicine - Concepts and Clinical Practice. 8th edition. 2013. Chapter 171: Cardiac Disorders. 2147.*

#32

In the above infant with cyanosis due to a presumed cardiac etiology, you have reached the maximum dose of PGE-1 without any effect. What congenital heart defect lesions causing cyanosis could cause a lack of response to PGE1?

(Choose two answers.)

    A. Tetralogy of Fallot

    B. Tricuspid Atresia

    C. Truncus Arteriosus

    D. Total Anomalous Pulmonary Venous Return

    E. Pulmonary Atresia

#32

Answer: C and D

There are two non-ductal dependent lesions: Truncus Arteriosus and TAPVR that may be responsible for this lack of response. However, these two defects cause less than 2% of cyanotic CHD, and PGE1 is a life-saving treatment for the vast majority of patients. If acute worsening occurs on PGE-1 an emergent echocardiogram should be performed. Early in the course of treatment the pediatric intensive care team should be consulted.

- *Rosen's Emergency Medicine - Concepts and Clinical Practice. 8th edition. 2013. Chapter 171: Cardiac Disorders. 2147-2151.*

#33

Which of the following congenital heart disease lesions often present in the first 3 weeks of life with shock and are ductal-dependent (need the ductus to deliver blood to the systemic circulation)?

(Choose three answers.)

    A. VSD

    B. Hypoplastic left heart syndrome (HLHS)

    C. ASD

    D. Critical aortic stenosis

    E. Coarctation of the aorta

#33

Answer: B, D, and E

In utero, these three lesions cause significant obstruction to normal blood flow, and the ductus is used for blood flow to the body. For example, in the fetus with coarctation of the aorta, a flange of tissue obstructs blood flow through the aorta. The patent ductus arteriosus allow blood to flow from the pulmonary artery through the ductus to the aorta and the body. After birth, when the ductus closes, systemic blood flow is dramatically decreased, and these lesions typically present in the newborn period in the first 3 weeks. HLHS is the most common deadly defect in the neonatal period and always presents with shock.

- *Rosen's Emergency Medicine - Concepts and Clinical Practice. 8th edition. 2013. Chapter 171: Cardiac Disorders. 2147-2151.*

#34

A child with known Tetralogy of Fallot (TOF) presents with a tet spell or cyanotic episode. She is cyanotic, tachypneic, irritable, and crying. What measures can be attempted?

A. Supplemental oxygen

B. Morphine

C. 20 cc/kg fluid bolus

D. Phenylephrine

E. Propranolol

F. All of the above

#34

Answer: F

Supplemental oxygen may assist in dilating the pulmonary vasculature. Morphine can also dilate the pulmonary vasculature. A 20 cc/kg bolus may improve preload and improve right ventricular filling. The parent should hold the infant over his shoulder with the infant's knees bent to increase systemic vascular resistance and to improve venous return to the heart. If the symptoms do not resolve, then phenylephrine may be used to increase systemic blood pressure to reverse the shunt. Propranolol can also be given to improve symptoms by relaxing the right ventricular outflow obstruction.

• *Rosen's Emergency Medicine - Concepts and Clinical Practice. 8th edition. 2013. Chapter 171: Cardiac Disorders. 2149-2151.*

#35

You are seeing a child with what seems like a nurse-maid's elbow (radial head subluxation). Which of the following procedures can be used to treat this?

(Choose two answers.)

    A. Supination/flexion

    B. Internal rotation

    C. External rotation

    D. Hyperpronation

    E. Hyperextension

Amy Kaji

#35

Answer: A and D

With the supination/flexion method, grasp the elbow with the thumb over the region of the radial head. Then, place the other hand on the wrist, and gently apply traction before supination. Supinate the forearm fully and then flex the elbow, all in one motion. With the hyperpronation method, the examiner grasps the child's upper arm, with the elbow flexed. With the other hand, the examiner rapidly pronates the arm at the wrist. A sudden release of resistance accompanied by a palpable click signifies reduction, but this may not always be present. Both methods of reduction are effective although the hyperpronation method may have greater rate of success. If reduction is achieved clinically and maintained, analgesics and follow-up visits are unnecessary. However, explain to the parent that there is a risk of repeat subluxation. Parents should use caution when holding the child by the hand and avoid twisting movements of the arm.

• *Harwood-Nuss' Clinical Practice of Emergency Medicine 5th edition. 2010. Chapter 265: Nursemaid's elbow. 1296-1297.*

#36

You are seeing a 17 year old with severe developmental delay who complains of fever, vomiting, and headache. Of note, he has a Ventriculoperitoneal Shunt (VP shunt) that has warranted 3 revisions, with the last one 4 months ago. Which of the following are FALSE about shunt malfunction?

A. There is a 40% incidence of malfunction in the first year after insertion.

B. Shunt fracture usually occurs within days after insertion, and the most common location is at the abdomen.

C. Shunt malfunction can occur due to ascites.

D. Shunt malfunction/migration can cause visceral perforation.

E. Shunt malfunction can be due to an infectious etiology.

#36

Answer: B

The Shunt Design Trial and Endoscopic Shunt Insertion Trial found up to 40% incidence of malfunction in the first year and 50% incidence by the second year following initial insertion. As the patient grows, there is increased tension and degradation on a system designed for a certain size and age. Thus, there is a greater likelihood of disconnection or fracture of the apparatus.

Shunt fracture usually occurs LATE (years after insertion), and the most common location along the shunt is near the clavicle or adjacent to the lower ribs. In contrast, disconnection, migration, and displacement occur EARLY, and obstruction can occur at any point.

Shunt malfunction may arise due to abdominal complications such as ascites, or an abdominal pseudocyst in proximity to the distal peritoneal catheter. The distal portion of a CSF shunt can also migrate and cause visceral damage and perforation. According to the Shunt design trial, 8.1% of shunt failures had an infectious etiology, and early shunt infections are due to Staph epidermidis and Staph aureus. Late infections may be due to gram negative organisms from the abdomen.

- Roberts and Hedges' Clinical Procedures in Emergency Medicine. 6th edition. 2013. Chapter 59: Management of Increased Intracranial Pressure and Intracranial Shunts. 1212-1217.

- Drake JM, et al. Randomized trial of cerebrospinal fluid shunt valve design in pediatric hydrocephalus. Neurosurgery. 1998 Aug;43(2):294-303; discussion 303-5.

#37

Some clinical features of VP shunt malfunction include which of the following:

A. Raised intracranial pressure – headaches and vomiting

B. Drowsiness

C. Decreased level of consciousness

D. Irritability

E. All of the above

#37

Answer: E

Common features include new onset nausea and vomiting (PPV 79%), irritability (PPV 78%), decreased level of consciousness (PPV 100%), lethargy, confusion, and headache. Uncommon features include increased seizure activity, diplopia, weakness, and visual disturbances. Possible clinical signs of malfunction include change in orbito-frontal circumference, and bulging fontanelle (PPV = 92%). Possible neurological signs include papilledema, cranial nerve palsies (specifically CN VI or CN IV), hyperactive reflexes and lower extremity hypertonia, a positive Babinski, and ataxic gait.

• *Roberts and Hedges' Clinical Procedures in Emergency Medicine. 6th edition. 2013. Chapter 59: Management of Increased Intracranial Pressure and Intracranial Shunts. 1212-1217.*

• *Drake JM, et al. Randomized trial of cerebrospinal fluid shunt valve design in pediatric hydrocephalus. Neurosurgery. 1998 Aug; 43(2):2 94-303; discussion 303-5.*

#38

Regarding VP shunt malfunction, which of the following is TRUE?

(Choose two answers.)

    A. CT scan is 100% sensitive for diagnosis.

    B. Shunt series is highly sensitive for the diagnosis.

    C. Pumping the shunt reservoir can ascertain whether there is a proximal or distal malfunction with 100% sensitivity and specificity.

    D. Shunt aspiration or tap should be performed by a neurosurgeon.

    E. Shunt malfunction signs and symptoms can be nonspecific.

#38

Answer: D and E

Estimates of CT sensitivity range from 64 to 94%, while the shunt series' sensitivity can be as low as 20% with a negative predictive value of 22%. CSF shunt malfunction can and often will present without ventriculomegaly. Despite the low sensitivity of the shunt series, studies have shown that it may aid in diagnosing a malfunction that was missed with the CT scan. When a shunt series and CT scan are performed, the combined sensitivity is 88% for detecting malfunctions.

Still, the present consensus is to obtain a shunt series, a head CT, and neurosurgical evaluation even if imaging is unremarkable, if malfunction is suspected. Shunt aspiration or tap should be performed, in general, only by a neurosurgeon. In the event of acute severe obstruction, shunt aspiration may be used to relieve symptoms in conjunction with acetazolamide, dexamethasone, and hyperventilation. Note that shunt malfunction signs and symptoms can be nonspecific.

. *Roberts and Hedges' Clinical Procedures in Emergency Medicine. 6th edition. 2013. Chapter 59: Management of Increased Intracranial Pressure and Intracranial Shunts. 1212-1217.*

#39

A seven year-old boy from El Salvador is brought to the ED for one month of anorexia, fatigue, and weight loss. According to the mom, the child only wants to eat salty foods. An outside clinic physician refers him to your hospital, because the child has a positive PPD and was found to have postural hypotension on examination. On his chemistry panel, which of the following would you NOT expect to see?

A. Hyponatremia

B. Hyperkalemia

C. Hypernatremia

D. High hematocrit

E. Hypoglycemia

#39

Answer: C

This unfortunate boy has B symptoms, salt-craving, and a positive PPD, all worrisome for adrenal insufficiency caused by a tuberculous. Tuberculosis is the most common cause of primary adrenal insufficiency worldwide. In contrast, the most common cause of primary adrenal insufficiency in the U.S. is Addison's disease. Adrenal insufficiency is characterized by insidious symptoms of weight loss, fatigue, anorexia, salt craving and postural hypotension. Causes of primary adrenal insufficiency (affecting the adrenals) include congenital adrenal hyperplasia, autoimmune disease, tuberculosis, meningococcal septicemia, adrenal infarction (Friderichsen-Waterhouse), and X-linked adrenoleukodystrophy. Causes of secondary adrenal insufficiency (affecting the HPA axis) include steroid therapy, pituitary or hypothalamic tumors, CNS surgery or radiation, or congenital hypopituitarism. Blood chemistry can show: hyponatremia, hyperkalemia, hypoglycemia, and hemoconcentration. Acute treatment includes volume resuscitation and 1-2 mg/kg IV hydrocortisone.

- *Rosen's Emergency Medicine - Concepts and Clinical Practice. 8th edition. 2013. Chapter 128: Thyroid and Adrenal Disorders. 1689.*

#40

You are caring for an 18 month old girl with a tracheostomy on home oxygen and chronic respiratory care. TRUE statements about pediatric tracheostomy related complications include which of the following?

(Choose two answers.)

A. Most pediatric tracheostomy-related complications occur outside the hospital setting.

B. The tracheostomy tube should extend 2 cm beyond the stoma and 5 cm beyond the carina.

C. Tracheostomy decannulation or dislodgement tends to occur more commonly in infants.

D. Tracheostomy obstruction tends to occur in older ventilated children.

E. A tracheostomy infection can present with tracheitis.

#40

Answer: A and E

Most pediatric tracheostomy-related complications occur outside the inpatient hospital setting. Thus, emergency physicians should be prepared to change a tube in the event of airway compromise. Choosing the appropriate diameter, length, and curvature of the tube is important when changing a tracheostomy tube because these factors will determine the effectiveness of the new airway.

According to the American Thoracic Society, the tube should extend 2 cm beyond the stoma but no further than 1-2 cm beyond the carina. Obstruction is one of the most common causes of malfunction. In children older than 1 year, the incidence is 14%, but it is higher in premature babies and newborns (72%) because of relatively smaller sized tubes in infants. The incidence of decannulation and dislodgement is more common in older ventilated children. Basically, obstruction is more common in young infants and decannulation is more common in older children. Tracheostomy infections commonly present with copious, yellow-green malodorous secretions, and it may progress to tracheitis.

- Sherman JM, et al. American Thoracic Society Care of the child with a chronic tracheostomy. American Journal of Respiratory and Critical Medicine. 2000; 161: 297-308.

#41

The 18 month old female with the tracheostomy is sitting in your ED with what appears to be copious, bright red bleeding from the tracheostomy site. What should you do?

A. Start antibiotics

B. Panic

C. Remove the tube

D. Deflate the cuff

E. Apply pressure to the bleeding site and inflate the cuff

#41

Answer: E

The mucosa adjacent to the tracheostomy site, the tracheostomy tip, and cuff is prone to pressure and irritation. With poor humidification, this mucosa becomes vulnerable to bleeding and subsequent granuloma formation. In the weeks following tracheostomy placement, granulomas may be soft and fragile but may become fibrous over time. Large granulomas may obstruct the lumen and increase the likelihood of bleeding. Chronic erosion of the anterior tracheal mucosa leads to the risk of communication with the innominate artery, resulting in massive, life-threatening bleeding. In these circumstances, treat with humidified oxygen, suction, and intravenous fluids to replace losses and refrain from removing the tube in the unstable patient, as the airway may be lost. Instead, apply pressure to the bleeding site if it can be visualized, or inflate the cuff to provide a tamponade effect until definitive treatment is available. Any bleed ultimately will need to be investigated by bronchoscopy.

- Roberts and Hedges' Clinical Procedures in Emergency Medicine. 6th edition. 2013. Chapter 7: Tracheostomy Care.146-148.

#42

You are now seeing a 2 year old male who is brought in by his parents because his gastrostomy tube was dislodged. It apparently was placed 9 months ago, and the dislodgement occurred 30 minutes prior to arrival. You recall that you had seen this very same child 2 weeks ago for an obstructed tube. Regarding gastrostomy tubes and their complications, which of the following is TRUE?

A. There are six main types of gastrostomy tubes.

B. A foley catheter may be placed temporarily to maintain stoma patency.

C. There is strong evidence that Coca-Cola can remove obstructions.

D. If the tube is obstructed, an attempt should be made to clear it with a stylet.

E. A dislodged jejunal tube should be replaced by a subspecialist (surgeon or interventional radiology) responsible for its insertion.

#42

Answer: E

There are three main types of gastrostomy tubes:

1. The MIC with an inflatable balloon tube end
2. The Button (commonly a mushroom tip tube end)
3. The Malecot with a collapsible wings tube end

A foley catheter may be placed temporarily if the gastrostomy is long-term (has been in place for greater than 3 months) and the dislodgement is recent. There is no definitive evidence that carbonated sodas are more effective than water at removing G-tube obstructions. A stylet should never be used to clear an obstruction, as this may cause a blind perforation of the tubing beneath the skin.

In the perioperative period (up to 3 months), the management of tube dislodgement must be approached with extreme caution since the stomach may not have fully adhered to the anterior abdominal wall and is at risk of separation. Placement of a foley catheter or replacement G-tube may disrupt the fistulous tract and create a false lumen and should only be performed in consultation with the pediatric surgeon. Administration of feedings into a blindly inserted tube can cause life-threatening pneumoperitoneum. Thus, it is recommended that a pediatric surgery or gastroenterology consult be obtained prior to replacement attempt. Similarly, a dislodged jejunal tube should be replaced only by the subspecialist.

- *Roberts and Hedges' Clinical Procedures in Emergency Medicine. 6th edition. 2013. Chapter 40: Nasogastric and Feeding Tube Placement. 823.*

#43

You are now seeing a 5 year old with short-gut syndrome, who has a partially implantable central venous catheter in place for total parenteral nutrition (TPN). His mother has brought him in because they were unable to infuse the TPN and medications today. TRUE statements about managing problems with indwelling venous access devices include which of the following?

A. Thrombotic occlusions are the most common complications of these central venous catheters

B. Non-thrombotic occlusion management depends on which formulas or medications have been infused prior to the obstruction.

C. If there is evidence of catheter displacement or breakage, the catheter should be clamped proximal to the damaged segment.

D. Air embolism should be suspected in a patient who has a central catheter presenting with dyspnea, tachypnea and associated history of tubing that has remained unclamped.

E. All of the above

#43

Answer: E

Thrombotic occlusions are the most common complication and can usually be managed with alteplase AFTER ensuring there is no mechanical obstruction. There are four types of occlusions although management will be similar for all:

1. Fibrin tail or flap
2. Fibrin sheath or sleeve
3. Intraluminal obstruction
4. Mural thrombus

If there is any leakage of blood or fluid, a break should be suspected and the catheter should be immediately clamped proximal to the damaged segment to prevent further leakage or introduction of an air embolus. Although rare, the incidence of air embolism is highest with venous access devices during the initial placement.

Suspicious should be raised of an air embolism in any patient with a central line who presents with dyspnea, tachypnea, lightheadedness, chest pain, tachycardia, and hypotension. On examination, you may hear a mill-wheel murmur representing a large air bolus trapped within the right ventricle. Immediately provide 100% oxygen, clamp the catheter, and perform Durant's maneuver (placing the patient on the left side in Trendelenburg) to ensure that air in the right ventricle can collect and move away from the right ventricular outflow tract.

- *Roberts and Hedges' Clinical Procedures in Emergency Medicine. 6th edition. 2013. Chapter 24: Indwelling Vascular Devices: Emergency Access and Management. 449-450.*

#44

You suspect that a 5 week old male has hypertrophic pyloric stenosis. TRUE statements about this illness include which of the following?

    A. Girls are affected more commonly than boys.

    B. Ultrasound is the diagnostic modality of choice, and its accuracy is greater than 95%.

    C. The age of the child and the timing of vomiting provide important clues to the etiology.

    D. A, B, C

    E. B and C

#44

Answer: E

Boys are affected at four times the rate of girls. Ultrasound has a diagnostic accuracy greater than 95%. The classic finding is a thickened pylorus. Ultrasound has an accuracy of > 95%. Children may have reflux early in life but pyloric stenosis, symptoms do not begin until after 2 weeks of age as the pylorus thickens.

•   *Rosen's Emergency Medicine - Concepts and Clinical Practice. 8th edition. 2013. Chapter 172: Gastrointestinal Disorders. 2170-2172.*

#45

You are seeing a 4 year old patient with a vagal nerve stimulator (VNS). TRUE statements about this device include which of the following?

A. These are implantable devices used to treat intractable cancer pain.

B. It is implanted just under the skin of the humerus.

C. A magnet can be used to stop the stimulation by holding the magnet over the device.

#45

Answer: C

VNS are implantable devices used to prevent seizures. The VNS looks like a pacemaker and is implanted by a neurosurgeon just under the skin of the chest. The device can reduce seizure frequency up to 50% by stimulation of the left vagus nerve. There are constant intermittent pulsations delivered to the vagus nerve. Similar to a pacemaker, a magnet can affect the device and cause cessation of vagal stimulation when it remains held over the VNS. However, any seizing child should be treated with first priority at seizure control while maintaining the airway and continuing an assessment for other causes of seizure whether, traumatic, metabolic, infectious or toxicologic.

- *Rosen's Emergency Medicine - Concepts and Clinical Practice. 8th edition. 2013. Chapter 187: Evaluation of the Developmentally or Physically Disabled Patient. 2409.*

#46

You are trying to determine if a newly born infant requires resuscitation. The baby was delivered in the ED parking lot. You are speaking to the paramedics to guide them in the field. Which of the following questions are important to ask in order to guide resuscitation?

(Choose three answers.)

    A. Is this a term gestation?

    B. Did the mother use any illegal drugs?

    C. Is the baby crying?

    D. Is the baby male?

    E. Does the baby have good muscle tone?

#46

Answer: A, C, and E

If the answer to all 3 of these questions is "yes," then the baby does not need resuscitation and should not be separated from the mother. The baby should be dried, placed skin-to-skin with the mother, and covered with dry linen to maintain temperature.

- *Kattwinkel J, et al. Neonatal resuscitation: 2010 American heart association guidelines for cardiopulmonary resuscitation and emergency cardiovascular care. Pediatrics. 2010; 126(5):1400-1413. full text*

#47

Regarding the patient with meconium seen during delivery, which of the following should always be done?

A. Suction the oropharynx before delivery of the shoulders.

B. Intubate the patient and directly suction all of these babies.

C. Both of the above

D. Neither of the above

#47

Answer: D

Only depressed infants born to mothers with meconium-stained amniotic fluid are at increased risk to develop meconium aspiration syndrome.

The need for endotracheal intubation with tracheal suctioning after delivery of the infant should be made based on the vigor of the infant, rather than on the consistency of the meconium. Tracheal suctioning should be performed in any neonate with meconium stained fluid and:

1. Absent or depressed respiration,
2. Poor muscle tone
3. Heart rate less than 100 beats/minute.

• *Kattwinkel J, et al. Neonatal resuscitation: 2010 American heart association guidelines for cardiopulmonary resuscitation and emergency cardiovascular care. Pediatrics. 2010; 126(5): 1400-1413. full text*

#48

The goal oxygen saturation in babies being resuscitated at birth should be:

A. 100%

B. It depends on whether the baby is term or pre-term.

C. 65-70% within the first minute

#48

Answer: C

C is true, and blended oxygen is recommended. In general if blended oxygen is not available, then resuscitation should be initiated with air. If the baby is bradycardic after 90 seconds of resuscitation with a lower concentration of oxygen, then the concentration should be increased to 100% until recovery of a normal heart rate. If the infant remains apneic or gasping or if the heart rate remains < 100 per minute, then positive pressure ventilations should be started.

Although scary to see an infant with a oxygen saturation of 65% at birth, it may take up to 10 minutes for a newborn to reach 90% saturation. An easy way of remembering the increase in saturations is 5% point increase for each minute after birth.

The median saturations by minute of age for term infants:

1 min - 68%

2 min - 76%

3 min - 81%

4 min - 88%

5 min - 92%

6 min - 94%

7 min - 95 %

8 min - 96%

9 min - 97%

10 min - 97%

• Kattwinkel J, et al. Neonatal resuscitation: 2010 American heart association guidelines for cardiopulmonary resuscitation and emergency cardiovascular care. Pediatrics. 2010; 126(5): 1400-1413. full text

• Dawson JA, et al. Defining the reference range for oxygen saturation for infants after birth. Pediatrics. 2010 Jun; 125(6): e1340-7 full text

#49

Regarding chest compressions in the neonate, which of the following is TRUE?

(Choose two answers.)

- A. Chest compressions are indicated if the heart rate is < 60 bpm despite adequate ventilation.

- B. Compressions should be delivered in the upper third of the sternum.

- C. Either the 2 thumb-encircling hands technique or compression with 2 fingers with a second hand supporting the back may be used.

- D. Compression ratio should be 15:2.

#49

Answer: A and C

The 2 finger technique may be preferable when access to the umbilicus is required for insertion of a UV Catheter. Compressions to ventilations should be performed at a 3:1 ratio with 90 compressions and 30 breaths. This ratio should be used for neonatal resuscitation where compromise of ventilation is nearly always the primary cause. Only if a primary cardiac etiology is suspected, 15:2 or 30:2 ratio should be used.

- Kattwinkel J, et al. Neonatal resuscitation: 2010 American heart association guidelines for cardiopulmonary resuscitation and emergency cardiovascular care. Pediatrics. 2010; 126(5): 1400-1413. full text

#50
When should neonatal resuscitation be discontinued?

A. If the heart rate is undetectable for 3 minutes

B. If the baby is cold

C. Both of the above

D. Neither of the above

#50

Answer: D

In a newly born baby with no detectable heart rate, it is appropriate to consider stopping resuscitation if the heart rate remains undetectable for 10 minutes.

· *Kattwinkel J, et al. Neonatal resuscitation: 2010 American heart association guidelines for cardiopulmonary resuscitation and emergency cardiovascular care. Pediatrics. 2010; 126(5): 1400-1413. full text*

#51

Examples of when neonatal resuscitation is NOT likely to be successful include which of the following?

(Choose two answers.)

A. Gestational age of 26 weeks

B. Anencephaly

C. Birth weight of 600g

D. Trisomy 13

Amy Kaji

#51

Answer: B and D

When gestation, birth weight, or congenital anomalies are associated with almost certain early death or high morbidity, resuscitation is not indicated. Examples include extreme prematurity (age < 23 weeks or birth weight < 400g), anencephaly, and some major chromosomal abnormalities, such as trisomy 13.

- Kattwinkel J, et al. Neonatal resuscitation: 2010 American heart association guidelines for cardiopulmonary resuscitation and emergency cardiovascular care. Pediatrics. 2010; 126(5): 1400-1413. full text

#52

A neonate appears to have respiratory depression. Which of the following are potential considerations?

A. Naloxone

B. BVM

C. Intubation

D. Laryngeal Mask Airway (LMA)

E. All except A

#52

Answer: E

LMAs are effective for ventilating newborns weighing more than 2000 g or after 34 weeks. Naloxone is not recommended as part of initial resuscitative efforts in the delivery room for newborns with respiratory depression. Heart rate and oxygenation should be restored by supporting ventilation.

- *Kattwinkel J, et al. Neonatal resuscitation: 2010 American heart association guidelines for cardiopulmonary resuscitation and emergency cardiovascular care. Pediatrics. 2010; 126(5): 1400-1413. full text*

PROCEDURES

Amy Kaji

#1

When comparing ultrasound-guided peripheral vein access to traditional approaches in patients with difficult access, which of the following statements is TRUE?

Ultrasonographic-guided peripheral intravenous access is:

A. More successful than traditional "blind" techniques

B. Requires less time than traditional "blind" techniques

C. Decreases the number of percutaneous punctures when compared to traditional "blind" techniques

D. Improves patient satisfaction

E. All of the above

#1

Answer: E

Costantino TG, et al studied the use of ultrasound at 2 university hospitals. Success rate was greater for the ultrasonographic group (97%) versus control (33%), with a difference in proportions of 64% (95% CI 39% to 71%). The ultrasonographic group required less overall time, 13 minutes versus 30 minutes, (95% CI 0.8 to 25.6), less time to successful cannulation from first percutaneous puncture, 4 minutes versus 15 minutes (95% CI 8.2 to 19.4), and greater patient satisfaction -- 8.7 versus 5.7 (95% CI 1.82 to 4.29)-- than the traditional landmark approach.

- *LLSA 2007: Costantino TG, et al. Ultrasound-guided peripheral intravenous access versus traditional approaches in patients with difficult intravenous access. Ann Emerg Med. 2005; 46(5): 456-461. full text*

#2

During curved blade laryngoscopy, which of the following maneuvers was demonstrated in a cadaver model to best improves the laryngeal view?

 A. Bimanual laryngoscopy

 B. Cricoid pressure

 C. Backward, rightward, upward pressure (BURP)

 D. No manipulation

 E. None of the above

#2

Answer: A

This study demonstrated optimization of the laryngeal view with bimanual laryngoscopy, rather than with cricoid pressure or the BURP (backwards, upward, rightward pressure) maneuver.

- *LLSA 2008: Levitan RM, et al. Laryngeal view during laryngoscopy: a randomized trial comparing cricoid pressure, backward-upward-rightward pressure, and bimanual laryngoscopy. Ann Emerg Med. 2006; 47: 548-555.*

- *Airway Cam - Bimanual Laryngoscopy http://www.airwaycam.com/bimanual-laryngoscopy.html*

#3

True statements about significant retrobulbar hematomas include all of the following EXCEPT:

A. Signs and symptoms include eye pain, nausea, vomiting, decreased vision, diplopia, RAPD, and proptosis.

B. The retina can withstand ischemia for only 90 minutes.

C. Definitive treatment includes head elevation, mannitol, acetazolamide, and timolol.

D. Canthotomy is performed by incising the lateral canthus.

E. The inferior arm of the lateral canthus tendon is cut to release the globe during a cantholysis.

#3

Answer: C

Temporizing treatments for retrobulbar hematomas involves head of bed elevation, ice packs, mannitol, acetazolamide, and timolol, but definitive treatment is lateral canthotomy and cantholysis.

- *Roberts and Hedges' Clinical Procedures in Emergency Medicine. 6th edition. 2013. Chapter 62: Ophthalmologic, Otolaryngologic, and Dental Procedures. 1293-1295.*

Amy Kaji

#4

Regarding ultrasound terminology, which of the following pairs is matched INCORRECTLY?

A. **Echogenic** – the propensity to reflect ultrasound waves. The more echogenic a structure, the whiter or lighter gray it appears.

B. **Hyperechoic** – a black appearance – examples include the kidneys, the spleen, and the uterus.

C. **Anechoic** – a black appearance – examples include unclotted blood, bile, urine, ascites, and effusions.

D. **Hypoechoic** – a gray appearance – examples include the kidneys, the spleen, and the uterus.

E. **Edge artifact** – a shadow far-field from the edge of hyperechoic structures.

#4

Answer: B

Hyperechoic refers to a relatively white appearance, and examples include the diaphragm, the pericardium, and bones. These structures are also echogenic. All of the other pairs are correct.

- *Ihnatsenka B, Pierre Boezaart A, Ultrasound: Basic understanding and learning the language. Int J Shoulder Surg. 2010; 4(3): 55–62.*

- *Ultrasound Podcast - http://bit.ly/kaji-ultarsound-basics*

#5

You are seeing a patient who has sustained multiple facial lacerations and you would like to perform various facial nerve blocks. Which of the following statements are TRUE regarding these blocks?

A. For an infraorbital nerve block, an extraoral or intraoral approach may be taken.

B. For a mental nerve block, an intraoral or extraoral approach may be taken.

C. For the auricular block, the anesthetic will be injected into a diamond shape around the pinna.

D. All of the above

#5

Answer: D

Infraorbital block

The infraorbital foramen is located just inferior to the lower edge of the orbit, centered below the pupil. Both extraoral or intraoral approaches can be used. Before either approach, palpate the infraorbital foramen. For the intraoral approach, place one finger on the infraorbital foramen and retract the upper lip. Identify the first maxillary premolar, and insert the needle into the mucobuccal fold and advance 0.5 - 1 cm below the palpated infraorbital foramen injected 2-4 cc of 1% lidocaine.

Mental block

The mental foramen lies at the apex of the lower second premolar. Similarly to the infraorbital block, palpate the foramen and advance the needle in parallel to the alveolar ridge ensuring not to enter the foramen. Inject 2-4 cc of 1% lidocaine and massage into the foramen.

Auricular block

For the auricular block, enter the skin superiorly and infiltrate along the superior/anterior aspect, and then infiltrate along the superior/posterior aspect of the ear. Then, repeat the same injection paths superior/posterior, but inferior to the pinna. A total of 10 to 20 ml of anesthetic is injected in a diamond shape around the pinna (the nerves involved include the auriculotemporal nerve, the lesser occipital nerve, and the greater auricular nerve).

- *Roberts and Hedges' Clinical Procedures in Emergency Medicine. 6th edition. 2013. Chapter 30: Regional Anesthesia of the Head and Neck.*

- *NYSORA - Nerve Block Techniques http://bit.ly/kaji-facial-blocks*

#6

Which of the following statements regarding propofol is FALSE?

A. It decreases cerebral metabolism and oxygen demand.

B. One complication that may result is called propofol infusion syndrome (PIS).

C. PIS is indicated by hypokalemia and respiratory acidosis.

D. Risk factors for PIS include high doses for prolonged periods of time (>48 hrs).

E. PIS can lead to cardiovascular collapse and death.

#6

Answer: C

Due to its rapid onset and fast metabolism, propofol is popular for emergency department sedation, especially in patients with traumatic brain injury (TBI). Propofol decreases cerebral metabolism and oxygen demand, and thus is believed to be neuroprotective. However, little data has demonstrated its benefit in lowering ICP. Prolonged use (>48 hrs) and large doses (> 4-5 mg/kg/hr) increase the risk for propofol infusion syndrome (PIS), which can result in heart failure, rhabdomyolysis, metabolic acidosis, acute renal failure, and cardiovascular collapse. Although first identified in children, PIS can occur in adults, as well.

• *Rosen's Emergency Medicine - Concepts and Clinical Practice. 8th edition. 2013. Chapter 4: Procedural Sedation and Analgesia. 58.*

• *Kam PC, Cardone D. Propofol infusion syndrome. Anaesthesia. 2007; 62(7): 690-701.*

• *Tobias JD, Leder M. Procedural sedation: A review of sedative agents, monitoring, and management of complications. Saudi J Anaesth. 2011 Oct;5(4):395-410. full text*

#7

You are seeing a 5 year old patient in whom you are considering suturing a laceration with absorbable plain gut versus nonabsorbable nylon sutures. If you repair with absorbable suture, what is the most likely outcome?

A. Worse cosmetic outcome

B. Increased chance of dehiscence

C. Increased wound infection

D. Benefit of not requiring suture removal

E. Greater need for scar revision

#7

Answer: D

Karounis H, et al. conducted a pediatric emergency department (1999-2001) trial where patients 1-18 years of age with lacerations < 12 hours old were randomized into two groups:

1. Those receiving absorbable plain gut sutures (group A)
2. Those receiving non-absorbable nylon sutures (group NA)

Exclusion criteria were: wounds that could be approximated by tissue adhesives, animal/human bites, gross contamination, puncture/crush wounds, wounds crossing joints, lacerations of tendon/nerve/cartilage, collagen vascular disease, immunodeficiency, diabetes mellitus, bleeding disorder, and scalp lacerations.

All wounds were reevaluated within ten days by a single research nurse who assessed the wounds using a previously validated wound evaluation score (WES). The patients were then seen by a single blinded plastic surgeon at four months who evaluated the wound for cosmesis.

At the short term follow up visit, no difference was found in the proportion of optimal WES scores between group A (63% of patients) and group NA (49% of patients) (relative risk = 0.73; 95% confidence interval [95% CI] = 0.45 to 1.17) or the rate of infection or dehiscence. At four month follow up, no differences were found in WES score between group A (36% of patients) and group NA (28% of patients) (relative risk = 0.88; 95% CI = 0.62 to 1.26).

- *Karounis H, et al. A randomized controlled trial comparing long-term cosmetic outcomes of traumatic pediatric lacerations repaired with absorbable plain gut versus nonabsorbable nylon sutures. Acad Emerg Med. 2004; 11(7): 730-735.*

#8

Cardiac tamponade is a state of hemodynamic compromise resulting from cardiac compression by fluid trapped in the pericardial space. Regarding the clinical presentation of cardiac tamponade, which of the following features is not found in the majority of patients with tamponade?

A. Dyspnea

B. Tachycardia

C. Elevated jugular venous pressure

D. Distant heart sounds

E. Pulsus paradoxus

#8

Answer: D

Roy CL, et al conducted a systematic review of the literature to determine the accuracy of history, physical exam, and basic diagnostic tests for the diagnosis of cardiac tamponade. Of the studies included, five features occur in the majority of patients with tamponade:

1. Dyspnea (sensitivity range, 87%-89%)
2. Tachycardia (sensitivity, 77%; 95% CI, 69%-85%),
3. Pulsus paradoxus (pooled sensitivity, 82%; 95% CI, 72%-92%),
4. Elevated jugular venous pressure (sensitivity, 76%; 95% CI, 62%-90%)
5. Cardiomegaly on chest radiograph (sensitivity, 89%; 95% CI, 73%-100%)

One study demonstrated the presence of pulsus paradoxus greater than 10 mm Hg in a patient with a pericardial effusion increases the likelihood of tamponade (likelihood ratio, 3.3; 95% CI, 1.8-6.3), while a pulsus paradoxus of 10 mm Hg or less greatly lowers the likelihood (likelihood ratio, 0.03; 95% CI, 0.01-0.24).

The above physical findings are useful for determining patients with cardiac tamponade, although they will be absent in some patients. Ultrasound findings such as right ventricular collapse, which was not assessed in this review, may offer even greater sensitivity.

- *LLSA 2009: Roy CL, et al. Does this patient with a pericardial effusion have cardiac tamponade? JAMA. 2007 Apr 25; 297(16): 1810-8. full text*

PSYCHIATRY

#1

Regarding schizophrenia, which of the following statements is FALSE?

A. Diagnostic features of schizophrenia include auditory hallucinations and delusions.

B. The lifetime risk of suicide is about 10% among patients with schizophrenia.

C. Administration of first-generation antipsychotic drugs such as haloperidol results in an blockade of dopamine D2 receptors.

D. Clozapine's main adverse side effect is its tendency to prolong the QT interval.

E. First-generation antipsychotic agents administered as a depot injection, despite the risk of tardive dyskinesia, remain the optimal therapy for patients who have a relapse because of poor adherence to a regimen of oral medication.

#1

Answer: D

Clozapine is the first atypical antipsychotic drug, and was marketed as having superior efficacy at decreasing psychotic features without the adverse effects on movement of the first-generation drugs. However, its major serious side effect is agranulocytosis. Patients taking clozapine must undergo frequent monitoring of the leukocyte count (weekly for the first six months and every two weeks thereafter, including the first four weeks after the patient has discontinued the drug). The incidence of agranulocytosis is 0.39% and the death rate among patients who take clozapine is 0.013%. Thus, the drug should not be given to patients with poor followup.

Other side effects include myocarditis and decreased seizure threshold. Clozapine reduces suicidal behavior and may be efficacious in patients who have failed all other antipsychotic therapy.

. *Freedman R. Schizophrenia. N Engl J Med. 2003 Oct 30; 349(18): 1738-49. full text*

#2

A 59-year-old woman, who describes herself as a lifetime "worrier" and has a family history of depression, reports having restless sleep, muscle tension, and fatigue. Recently, her anxiety has intensified about her children, her job, and her health, and it is having a negative effect on her family and work life. Regarding the clinical entity of generalized anxiety disorders, which of the following statements is FALSE?

- A. Anxiety disorders are the most prevalent psychiatric conditions in the United States aside from disorders involving substance abuse.

- B. In evaluating patients for generalized anxiety disorder, be sure to consider medical conditions, illegal drug use, drug withdrawal, and both prescribed and over-the-counter medications.

- C. Factors suggesting an organic cause for anxiety include an onset of the symptoms after the age of 35 years, no personal or family history of anxiety, no increase in stress, and a poor response to anti-anxiety medication.

- D. The most extensively studied psychotherapy for anxiety is psychodynamic, Freudian-based therapy.

- E. For generalized anxiety alone or anxiety that is associated with depression, a reasonable first-line approach is to administer an SSRI.

#2

Answer: D

The most extensively studied psychotherapy for anxiety is cognitive behavioral therapy. This therapy, which teaches patients to substitute positive thoughts for anxiety-provoking ones, usually involves 6 to 12 individual weekly sessions. Sessions include diary tracking of feelings, role playing, and rehearsed responses to difficult situations.

In one randomized, controlled study, 32% of patients in the group that received cognitive behavioral therapy had clinically significant improvement at three months, and 42% had clinically significant improvement at six months. No one in the control group, had improvement at 3 months. Following patients for 8-14 years in another randomized trial demonstrated that in patients who had an initial improvement, 50% remained improved.

. *LLSA 2007: Fricchione G. Generalized anxiety disorder. N Eng J Med. 2004 Aug 12;351(7):675-82.*

#3

Regarding the undifferentiated agitated patient that presents to the ED, which of the following statements are TRUE?

(Choose three answers.)

A. Practitioners generally should rule out a psychiatric cause of agitation first.

B. Physicians should always check both an oxygen saturation and a finger-stick glucose level.

C. Approaching any agitated patient, especially one considered to be at high risk for violence should be done with safety of the ED staff in mind.

D. Once an agitated patient arrives in the ED, all efforts should be made to ensure that the patient is physically comfortable.

E. For patients whose behavior continues to escalate and refuse medication, continued discussion and hypnosis is recommended.

#3

Answer: B, C, and D

Although it isn't always easy to distinguish between agitation of psychiatric and medical origin, practitioners should generally rule out organic causes of delirium first before assuming that the agitation is psychiatric in etiology. Easily correctable causes such as hypoxia and hypoglycemia should be assessed early in the patient's care. Always ensure that the ED staff is safe whenever approaching an agitated patient. Also, move the patient away from other patients. Remove all potential weapons and sharp instruments. For patients whose behavior continues to worsen, forceful restraint is recommended and IM or IV medication should assist in the restraint. Setting limits with the patient upfront can defuse a potentially hostile situation and can often be accomplished by bargaining with food and drink. Assure that the location of the patient is quiet and away from agitating sounds or chaos of the ED.

- *Rosen's Emergency Medicine - Concepts and Clinical Practice. 8th edition. 2013. Chapter 188: The Combative Patient.*

#4

Regarding the use of haloperidol for the chemical restraint of the undifferentiated agitated patient, which of the following statements is TRUE?

(Choose two answers.)

A. Often causes hypotension

B. Often causes respiratory depression

C. Carries a black-box warning about the risks of using it to treat psychosis

D. Can cause dystonic and other extrapyramidal reactions

E. It has potent anticholinergic activity

#4

Answer: C and D

Haloperidol (a high potency typical antipsychotic) has a number of properties that make it attractive for use in the emergency department. It also has minimal anticholinergic activity and little interactions with other non-psychiatric medications. Time to onset is within 30 minutes and re-dosing can occur every hour. Typical initial doses are 5 mg. Haloperidol carries a black-box warning about the risks of using it to treat dementia-related psychosis. It lengthens QT intervals and should be used cautiously in patients whose intervals are already prolonged or who are taking other QT prolonging drugs. Because of its action at the D2 receptor in the basal ganglia, haloperidol can cause dystonic and extrapyramidal reactions. Benadryl administration along with the haloperidol can minimize the extrapyramidal effects. It has a long record of safety in the ED and if the patient becomes over sedated, it does not depress respiratory drive or cause hypotension.

- *Rosen's Emergency Medicine - Concepts and Clinical Practice. 8th edition. 2013. Chapter 188: The Combative Patient. 2417.*

#5

The goal of treating acute agitation in the ED includes all of the following EXCEPT:

A. Inducing sleep in the patient

B. Protecting and calming the patient

C. Protecting and calming the staff

D. Allowing the patient's participation in guiding care to whatever extent possible

#5

Answer: A

Many emergency physicians and staff think that the only properly sedated patient is one who is sleeping. Current guidelines on sedation state that the proper goal of sedation is to calm patients and reduce the risk of violence, while still allowing them to participate in their own care as much as possible. More practically, however, patients who are not asleep are easier to obtain a disposition from the emergency department. Sleeping patients cannot be evaluated by consultants and have increased lengths of stay. Some research indicated that both waiting room times and length of stay for all ED patients increase in a step-wise fashion as the number of psychiatric holds in the ED increases.

- *Rosen's Emergency Medicine - Concepts and Clinical Practice. 8th edition. 2013. Chapter 188: The Combative Patient. 2414-2421.*

#6

You are seeing a patient with schizophrenia who has a necrotizing infection of his left hand that will need surgery. He, however, refuses treatment. In psychiatric patients, what is the strongest predictor of decisional incapacity?

A. Dementia

B. Lack of insight (lack of awareness of illness)

C. Being depressed

D. Being on medications

E. Age

#6

Answer: B

Among psychiatric disorders, schizophrenia has a stronger association with impaired capacity than depression; roughly 50% of patients hospitalized with an acute episode of schizophrenia have impairment with regard to at least one element of capacity, as compared with 20 to 25% of patients admitted with depression. Among psychiatric patients, lack of insight (the lack of awareness of illness and the need for treatment) has been reported to be the strongest predictor of incapacity. Patients on psychiatric medications, regardless of age or comorbidities or other psychiatric illness such as depression, can still be capable of consenting for procedures.

Competence and capacity are often used interchangeably. Incompetence is a legal designation by a court where incapacity is a patient's inability to make decisions regarding their health care. Patients with capacity to make a decision should understand the options of treatment, the consequences of accepting or refusing treatment, and the costs and benefits regarding that treatment.

• Appelbaum PS. Assessment of Patients' Competence to Consent to Treatment. N Engl J Med. 2007; 357(18): 1834-1840.

• Rosen's Emergency Medicine - Concepts and Clinical Practice. 8th edition. 2013. Bioethics. e40.

PULMONARY

#1

Which of the following is NOT a limitation of the Pneumonia Patient Outcome Research Team (PORT) Pneumonia Severity Index scoring system?

    A. It does not include pulse oximetry in the initial determination of class I patients.

    B. Some patients with conditions (e.g., immunosuppression) that contribute to decision making are not included in the predictor variables.

    C. The dichotomous construction of some of the variables may oversimplify the physician's decisions.

    D. PORT was validated as a mortality prediction rule but NOT as a method of triaging patients with community acquired pneumonia.

    E. All of the above are true.

#1

Answer: E

All of the above statements are true. Limitations of the PORT PSI classification scheme include the following:

1. There may be medical and psychosocial contra-indications to outpatient care.

2. Some patients with conditions (eg, immunosuppression) that contribute to decision making are not included in the model's predictors.

3. The dichotomous construction of some of the variables may oversimplify the physician's decisions.

4. It does not include pulse oximetry in the initial determination of class I patients.

5. The physician's clinical judgment should supersede a strict application of this scoring system.

6. PORT was validated as a mortality prediction rule and not as a method for triage of patients with CAP.

• *Nazarian DJ, et al. Clinical Policy: Critical Issues in the Management of Adult Patients Presenting to the Emergency Department With Community-Acquired Pneumonia. Ann Emerg Med. 2009 Nov; 54(5):704-31. full text*

#2

Which of the following statements regarding magnesium is FALSE?

A. Magnesium is a physiologic regulator of intracellular calcium flux and is an effective bronchodilator.

B. Magnesium prevents histamine from mast cells and opposes the action of acetylcholine.

C. Magnesium inhibits bronchial smooth muscle contraction.

D. Both aerosolized and intravenous magnesium are FDA approved to treat patients with asthma for whom maximal standard therapy has failed.

E. Side effects of magnesium include hypotension.

#2

Answer: D

Although some studies demonstrate benefit, magnesium is not FDA approved for use in asthma. Bronchodilation is observed within 2 to 5 minutes. However, the effect disappears rapidly after treatment is discontinued so bronchodilators must always be paired with magnesium.

- *Rosen's Emergency Medicine - Concepts and Clinical Practice. 8th edition. 2013. Chapter 73: Asthma. 951.*

#3

Several asthma scoring indices have been proposed to predict the need for hospitalization in asthma, but all have proven disappointing. Which of the following patients is LEAST warranting of admission?

A. Patient whose condition deteriorates in the emergency department

B. Patient who has wheezing after three nebulizer treatments but has an oxygen saturation of 100% while ambulating with no increased work of breathing

C. Patient with paO_2 of less than 60 mm Hg, hypercapnia, and acidosis

D. Patients with a pretreatment FEV1 of less than 30% of predicted and a posttreatment FEV1 less than 50-60% predicted

E. Patients with abnormal vital signs

#3

Answer: B

Many patients with asthma will continue to have wheezing after treatments. Patients who improve enough to be discharged from the ED have residual airway obstruction for several weeks after the acute episode subsides. Therefore, arrangements must be made for ongoing treatment and early follow-up. A non-tapering 3 to 10 day course of oral corticosteroids and a beta agonist should be prescribed, and a chronic regimen of inhaled steroids or leukotriene inhibitor may be started as an outpatient.

- *Rosen's Emergency Medicine - Concepts and Clinical Practice. 8th edition. 2013. Chapter 73: Asthma. 952-955.*

#4

Proposed risk factors for primary spontaneous pneumothorax (PSP) include all of the following EXCEPT:

A. Smoking

B. Marfan's syndrome

C. Pregnancy

D. Family history

E. Homocystinuria

F. Thoracic endometriosis

#4

Answer: C

Smoking, Marfan's syndrome, family history of PSP, homocystinuria, and thoracic endometriosis are all thought to be risk factors for primary spontaneous pneumothorax. The subpleural blebs that predispose patients to primary spontaneous pneumothorax are probably due to airway inflammation resulting from cigarette smoking in many cases.

In an analysis of four studies that included 505 patients with PSP, 461 of the patients (91%) were smokers. The risk of PSP directly related to the amount of cigarette smoked. When compared to nonsmokers the risk of PSP was greater in light smokers (one to 12 cigarettes per day), 21 times higher in moderate smokers (13 to 22 cigarettes per day), and 102 times higher in heavy smokers (>22 cigarettes per day).

Reports have also described increased risk of PSP in families with prior PSP. There is also a phenomenon referred to as catamenial pneumothorax, where thoracic endometriosis causes PSP in women during menstruation.

- *Rosen's Emergency Medicine - Concepts and Clinical Practice. 8th edition. 2013. Chapter 77: Pleural Diseases. 988-992.*

Amy Kaji

#5

In contrast to primary spontaneous pneumothorax, a secondary spontaneous pneumothorax (SSP) is defined as a pneumothorax that occurs as a complication of underlying lung disease. True statements about SSP include all of the following EXCEPT:

A. Nearly every lung disease can be complicated by secondary spontaneous pneumothorax (SSP).

B. Symptoms due to SSP are generally less severe than those associated with primary spontaneous pneumothorax.

C. Persistent air leaks are more common and tend to persist longer when due to SSP, compared to primary spontaneous pneumothorax.

D. A pneumothorax may be difficult to distinguish from a large, thin-walled, air-containing bulla.

E. None of the above

#5

Answer: B

Symptoms due to SSP are generally more severe than with primary spontaneous pneumothorax, most likely due to the decreased pulmonary reserve in patient with SSP and underlying chronic lung disease. Any chronic lung disease can be complicated by SSP although it is most commonly associated with chronic obstructive pulmonary disease, pneumocystis jirovecii infection, cystic fibrosis, and tuberculosis. Hospitalization is recommended in patients with secondary spontaneous pneumothorax due to complicating comorbidities.

- *Rosen's Emergency Medicine - Concepts and Clinical Practice. 8th edition. 2013. Chapter 77: Pleural Diseases. 988-992.*

- *Sahn SA, Heffner JE. Spontaneous pneumothorax. N Engl J Med. 2000; 342(12): 868-74. full text*

#6

Regarding small pneumothoraces, which of the following plain radiograph positions is the most sensitive for detection?

A. Upright chest X-ray

B. Lateral decubitus

C. Supine film

D. Inspiratory X-ray

E. Expiratory X-ray

#6

Answer: B

In upright patients, the accumulation of gas occurs primarily in an apical lateral location. As little as 50 mL of pleural gas can be visible. The value of expiratory chest radiographs in detecting pneumothoraces has been grossly overstated. As an example, one study of 85 patients with pneumothoraces and 93 controls found that inspiratory and expiratory upright chest radiographs have equal sensitivity for pneumothorax detection. In supine patients, approximately 500 mL of pleural gas is needed for definitive diagnosis of a pneumothorax.

In theory, a small pneumothorax can be more easily detected in the lateral decubitus view. In this position, as little as 5 mL of pleural gas was visible on the non-dependent side, during a cadaver study of pneumothoraces. Ultrasound may offer even a more sensitive and specific means of detection in the hands of an experienced operator.

- Rosen's Emergency Medicine - Concepts and Clinical Practice. 8th edition. 2013. Chapter 77: Pleural Diseases. 988-992.

- Carr JJ, et al. Plain and computed radiography for detecting experimentally induced pneumothorax in cadavers: implications for detection in patients. Radiology. 1992 Apr; 183(1): 193-9.

- Seow, A, et al. Comparison of upright inspiratory and expiratory chest radiographs for detecting pneumothoraces. AJR. 1996 Feb; 166(2): 313-6.

#7

Mechanisms of cocaine-induced pulmonary injury include which of the following?

A. Barotrauma

B. Vasospasm

C. Inflammation due to inflammatory mediators

D. Cellular toxicity

E. All of the above

#7

Answer: E

Mechanisms of cocaine-induced pulmonary injury include barotrauma and vasospasm leading to ischemia. Prolonged vasospasm can result in ventilation-perfusion lung scan abnormalities that mimic a pulmonary embolism and can only be excluded by pulmonary angiography.

"Crack Lung" occurs within 48hrs of smoking cocaine and involves alveolar infiltrates, eosinophilia, and fever. A common practice among crack smokers is to perform a Valsalva maneuver after inhalation. This can also lead to the development of pneumothorax, pneumomediastinum, and pneumopericardium. Chronic cocaine exposure can also cause diffuse alveolar damage, diffuse alveolar hemorrhage, bronchiolitis obliterans with organizing pneumonia (BOOP), and interstitial pneumonitis. In addition, smoked cocaine can cause noncardiogenic pulmonary edema, pulmonary infarctions, and interstitial pulmonary fibrosis. It is speculated that these tissue alterations result from direct cellular toxicity, constriction of the pulmonary vasculature with resultant pulmonary ischemia. There has also been accounts of direct thermal injury to both upper and lower airways from crack cocaine.

- *Rosen's Emergency Medicine - Concepts and Clinical Practice. 8th edition. 2013. Chapter 154: Cocaine and Sympathomimetics. 1999-2002.*

Amy Kaji

#8

Most mediastinal tumors are asymptomatic and are discovered when CT scans and plain radiographs are ordered for other reasons. However, some tumors can cause symptoms, and these may include:

A. Dysphagia

B. Horner's syndrome

C. Paralysis

D. Elevated hemidiaphragm

E. All of the above

#8

Answer: E

Tumors in children are often symptomatic and may cause respiratory difficulty and recurrent pulmonary infections, while in adults, tumors are often found incidentally. Severe pain is typically a sign of advanced, invasive disease. Multiple signs and symptoms may arise due to involvement of different mediastinal or surrounding structures:

1. Airway compression can lead to recurrent pulmonary infection and/or hemoptysis.
2. Esophageal compression can cause dysphagia.
3. Involvement of the spinal column can result in paralysis.
4. Phrenic nerve damage can present with an elevated hemidiaphragm.
5. Hoarseness can occur due to recurrent laryngeal nerve involvement.
6. Horner's and superior vena cava syndromes arise due to sympathetic ganglion and superior vena caval involvement.
7. Mediastinal tumors are often associated with systemic diseases such as thymoma with myasthenia gravis, goiter with thyrotoxicosis, and parathyroid adenoma with hyperparathyroidism.

• *Shield's General Thoracic Surgery 7th edition, 2009. Primary Mediastinal Tumors and Symptoms Associated with Mediastinal Lesions. 2487-2491.*

Amy Kaji

#9

The most common cause of a transudative pulmonary effusion is:

    A. Hemothorax

    B. Congestive heart failure

    C. Cirrhosis

    D. Pulmonary embolism

    E. Renal failure

#9

Answer: B

The most common cause of a transudative pleural effusion is left ventricular failure. Pleural effusions related to left ventricular failure are most commonly bilateral. Other causes of transudative pleural effusions include constrictive pericarditis, hepatic cirrhosis, and renal failure.

The most common etiologies leading to an exudative effusion are empyema and malignancy.

- *Rosen's Emergency Medicine - Concepts and Clinical Practice. 8th edition. 2013. Chapter 77: Pleural Diseases. 992-996.*

#10

All of the following are causes of a hemothorax, EX-CEPT:

    A. Trauma

    B. Malignancy

    C. Pulmonary embolus

    D. Constrictive pericarditis

    E. Leaking aortic aneurysm

#10

Answer: D

A hemothorax is defined as a bloody pleural effusion with a hematocrit exceeding half the value in peripheral blood. It can be seen after trauma, pulmonary embolism, as a result of metastatic disease, after anticoagulant therapy, or as a sequela of a leaking aortic aneurysm.

- *Rosen's Emergency Medicine - Concepts and Clinical Practice. 8th edition. 2013. Chapter 77: Pleural Diseases. 993.*

#11

The two most common etiologies of a chylothorax are:

(Choose two answers.)

    A. Mediastinal lymphoma

    B. Mediastinal bronchogenic carcinoma

    C. Surgery

    D. Filariasis

    E. Congenital lymphatic duct obstruction

#11

Answer: A and B

Chylothorax is most often the result of mediastinal tumor involvement by lymphoma or bronchogenic carcinoma. These two neoplasms account for the majority of chylothoraces, while trauma, including damage during surgery, accounts for the remainder. Rare causes of chylothorax include filariasis, lymphangioleiomyomatosis, congenital anomalies of the thoracic duct, and idiopathic chylothorax. Disruption of the thoracic duct leads may lead to the formation of a chylous duct cyst that appears as a mediastinal mass until it perforates and causes a pleural effusion. A right sided chylothorax indicates lower third thoracic duct injury, while left sided chylothoraces indicate an injury located in the upper two thirds of the thoracic duct.

- *Shield's General Thoracic Surgery 7th edition, 2009. Anatomy of the Thoracic Duct and Chylothorax. 829.*

#12

Which of the following are potential complications from endotracheal intubation and ventilatory management?

A. Cardiac dysfunction and hypotension

B. Barotrauma and pneumothorax

C. Elevated intracranial pressure

D. Ventilator-induced lung injury

E. Auto-PEEP

F. All of the above

#12

Answer: F

Hypotension, barotrauma, and ventilator-associated lung injury (VALI) are major issues related to mechanical ventilation. Hypotension can result from decreased venous return from elevated intrathoracic pressure or from the sedation or associated hypovolemia prior to the intubation. Barotrauma results from elevated pulmonary pressures and can be avoided by using lower tidal volumes. Using lower tidal volumes will also decrease the risk of VALI. Pneumonia is a long-term potential complication of mechanical ventilation and can be reduced by elevating the patient's head 30 degrees or by using reverse Trendelenburg bed positioning.

- *Rosen's Emergency Medicine - Concepts and Clinical Practice. 8th edition. 2013. Chapter 2: Mechanical Ventilation and Noninvasive Ventilatory Support. 28-29.*

#13

You are seeing a 35 year old female non-smoking patient who presents with a dry cough and dyspnea on exertion for the last 3 months. She denies any orthopnea, but she is currently 91% on room air with a heart rate of 85 bpm. Her chest X-ray demonstrates what appears to be interstitial markings possibly consistent with pulmonary fibrosis and a questionable lung mass. Her creatinine is found to be 3.0 The best diagnostic test would be:

A. Repeat Chest X-ray

B. V/Q scan

C. High resolution non-contrast CT scan of chest

D. CT scan of chest with IV contrast

E. Ultrasound of chest

#13

Answer: C

High-resolution non-contrast computed tomography (HRCT) scan is regarded as the imaging modality of choice to evaluate patients with known or suspected interstitial lung disease, malignancies, and concerning lung masses. For this particular patient, contrast administration is relatively contraindicated because of her underlying renal dysfunction, and thus, a non-contrast test is preferred. Although tissue will later be required for final diagnosis the findings on CT will guide further inpatient management. Current CT technology allows for detailed assessment of interstitial compartments.

- *Sung A, et al. High-resolution chest tomography in idiopathic pulmonary fibrosis and interstitial pneumonia: utility and challenges. Curr Opin Pulm Med 2007; 13: 451-457.*

Amy Kaji

#14

You are seeing a 40 year old female patient who complains of sudden onset right sided pleuritic chest pain. She has no medical history and has no risk factors for pulmonary emboli. She states that she had a viral syndrome with cough, congestion and some diarrhea 3 days prior to the chest pain onset. On examination, she has a temperature of 100.8 °F (38 °C), with a heart rate of 90 beats per minute, oxygen saturation of 100%, and she is splinting during respirations. Her X-rays demonstrate some atelectasis, d-dimer is normal, and you suspect that she has pleurodynia.

TRUE statements about this disease process include which of the following?

(Choose three answers.)

A. Pleurodynia is most commonly caused by the Coxsackie B virus.

B. Pathophysiology demonstrates muscle necrosis of the intercostal muscles, and this often leads to an elevated CPK level.

C. The transmission is via respiratory droplet.

D. It is often associated with a fever, sore throat, and headache.

E. Treatment is based upon initiating acyclovir or valacyclovir within the first 24 hours of symptom onset.

#14

Answer: A, B, and D

Pleurodynia is primarily caused by Coxsackievirus B virus associated gastroenteric infection. The transmission is fecal-oral or hematogenous, and treatment is primarily based upon anti-inflammatory agents, such as ibuprofen. There is no role for anti-viral agents. The onset of chest pain is acute. During attacks, the pain is severe, intense, and excruciating, lasting seconds to a minute. The paroxysms are caused by intercostal muscle inflammation. The attacks of pain and shortness of breath can last for up to 3-5 days. However, there can be periods of relapses over the course of a month. Pleurodynia is also called Bornholm disease or the "devil's grippe."

- *Rosen's Emergency Medicine - Concepts and Clinical Practice. 8th edition. 2013. Chapter 130: Viral Illnesses. 1732.*

#15

Which of the following is NOT a cause of hypoxemia?

A. Hypoventilation

B. Low inspired oxygen

C. Right to left shunt

D. Ventilation-perfusion abnormality

E. Carbon monoxide poisoning

#15

Answer: E

In addition to hypoventilation, low inspired oxygen, right to left shunt, V/Q mismatch, and diffusion impairment is also a cause of hypoxemia. It is important to appreciate that hypoxemia refers to low partial pressure of oxygen in the blood and NOT low oxygen content of blood. Severe anemia, hemoglobinopathies, carbon monoxide poisoning, as well as histotoxic poisons such as cyanide, lead to TISSUE hypoxia and are NOT causes of hypoxemia. PaO_2 in these cases is normal. Specifically, with carbon monoxide poisoning, the PaO_2 will be normal but the oxygen carrying of the RBCs will be decreased. Also, remember that in a given patient, mixed causes of hypoxemia occur frequently and it is often impossible to define precisely the extent of the contribution of each mechanism in the acutely ill patient.

•   *Rosen's Emergency Medicine - Concepts and Clinical Practice. 8th edition. 2013. Chapter 159: Inhaled Toxins. 2041-2042.*

. *Prockop LD, Chichkova R. Carbon monoxide intoxication: an updated review. J Neurol Sci. 2007 Nov 15; 262(1-2): 122-30. full text*

#16

FALSE statements about the alveolar-arterial oxygen difference [P(A-a)O$_2$] include which of the following:

A. In a young adult breathing room air (FiO$_2$ 21%), the normal P(A-a)O$_2$ is about 10-12.

B. The gradient exists partially due to venous admixture from a portion of the bronchial circulation venous blood drains into the pulmonary vein.

C. The gradient exists partially due to venous admixture from a portion of the coronary circulation venous blood draining through the thebesian veins into the left ventricle.

D. The normal P(A-a)O$_2$ decreases with age.

E. The change in the gradient with age reflects the change in V/Q with age.

#16

Answer: D

The normal range for $P(A-a)O_2$ increases with age. The formula is A-a gradient = (Age/4) +4. The increase is due to the age-dependence of normal PaO2. PaO_2 declines slightly over the years and reflects the change in VA/Q ratio of the aging lungs. At age 80, the normal A-a gradient is 24.

A-a $_{O2}$ Gradient = (Fi_{O2}) * (Atmospheric Pressure - H_2O Pressure) - $(Pa_{CO2}/0.8)$

- Harris EA, et al. The normal alveolar-arterial oxygen tension gradient in man. Clin Sci Mol Med. 1974 Jan; 46(1): 89-104.

- MD Calc http://www.mdcalc.com/a-a-o2-gradient/#about-calc

#17

True or False: A chest radiograph should be obtained on all patients with an acute asthma exacerbation.

A. True

B. False

#17

Answer: B

A chest radiograph is of little value in most acute asthma exacerbations and its use should be restricted to patients thought to have a complicating cardiopulmonary process, such a pneumonia, pneumothorax, pneumomediastinum, or congestive heart failure. Patients who do not respond to optimal therapy and require hospital admission have a higher likelihood of radiographically identifiable, unsuspected, clinically significant pulmonary complications of asthma (15% among asthmatics).

- *Rosen's Emergency Medicine - Concepts and Clinical Practice. 8th edition. 2013. Chapter 73: Asthma. 947-948.*

#18

The most common cause of small-volume hemoptysis is:

A. Bronchitis

B. Tuberculosis pneumonia

C. Cancer

D. Cystic fibrosis

E. Arteriovenous malformation

#18

Answer: A

Hemoptysis is defined as the expectoration of blood from the respiratory tract that originates below the vocal cords. Most cases are mild and consist of blood-tinged sputum. The most common cause is bronchitis. Rarely, hemoptysis is accompanied by massive blood loss, generally defined as 100 to 600 ml of blood over a 24 hour period. Only 1-5% of hemoptysis patients have massive or life-threatening hemorrhage; worldwide, TB and bronchiectasis are responsible for most cases. In developed nations, however, cancer, cystic fibrosis, arteriovenous malformations, and post-procedural bleeding are more common.

- *Rosen's Emergency Medicine - Concepts and Clinical Practice. 8th edition. 2013. Chapter 24: Hemoptysis. 203-205.*

#19

You are seeing a patient with a history of COPD, who presents with an exacerbation. You are debating whether to give him steroids and the best route. TRUE statements about treatment of COPD include which of the following?

(Choose three answers.)

    A. The mainstays of acute exacerbation of COPD include supplemental oxygen, short acting bronchodilators, and systemic corticosteroid.

    B. Treatment failure is lower for oral steroids than intravenous steroids.

    C. Oral treatment has not been shown to be worse than intravenous treatment.

    D. The benefit of steroids is clear, and the optimal route is via nebulization for the acute exacerbation of COPD.

#19
Answer: A, B, and C

A cohort study at 414 US hospitals examined the use of systemic corticosteroids during the first 2 hospital days in patients admitted to a non-intensive care setting.

The outcome was a composite measure of treatment failure (requiring mechanical ventilation), inpatient mortality, or readmission for acute exacerbation of COPD within 30 days of discharge, length of stay and hospital costs.

Of a total 79,985 patients, 73,765 (92%) were initially treated with intravenous steroids, whereas 6220 (8%) received oral treatment.

1.4% (95% CI, 1.3%-1.5%) of the intravenous group and 1.0% (95% CI, 0.7%-1.2%) of the orally treated patients died during hospitalization.

10.9% (95% CI, 10.7%-11.1%) of the intravenously and 10.3% (95% CI, 9.5%-11.0%) of the orally treated patients experienced the composite outcome.

After multivariable adjustment, including the propensity for oral treatment, the risk of treatment failure among patients treated orally was not worse than for those treated intravenously (odds ratio [OR], 0.93; 95% CI, 0.84-1.02). In a propensity-matched analysis, the risk of treatment failure was significantly lower among orally treated patients (OR, 0.84; 95% CI, 0.75-0.95), as was length of stay and cost.

- *Lindenauer PK, et al. Association of corticosteroid dose and route of administration with risk of treatment failure in acute exacerbation of COPD. JAMA. 2010; 303: 2359-2367. full text*

Amy Kaji

#20

Regarding community acquired pneumonia, which of the following statements is TRUE?

A. It is the 7th leading cause of death in the US.

A. It is the 7th leading cause of death in the US.

B. Pneumonia mortality rates have decreased significantly since penicillin became routinely available.

C. Health-care associated pneumonia is defined as infection occurring within 180 days of a 2 day or longer hospitalization

D. CURB-65 is a severity of illness scores which predicts mortality, using features of age ≥65, confusion, urea, respiratory rate, and base deficit.

E. Pneumonia severity index stratifies patients into 5 categories based on mortality risk, and groups I and II should be treated in the ICU.

#20

Answer: A

Pneumonia is the 7th leading cause of death, and it carries an age-adjusted mortality rate up to 22%. Despite clinical advances, pneumonia mortality rates have not decreased significantly since penicillin became routinely available.

There are 4 categories of pneumonia

1. Community Acquired Pneumonia (CAP)
2. Hospital-acquired pneumonia (HAP)
3. Ventilator-associated pneumonia (VAP)
4. Health-care associated pneumonia (HCAP).

CAP is defined as an acute pulmonary infection in a patient who is not hospitalized or living in a long-term care facility 14 or more days before presentation and does not meet criteria for HCAP. HCAP is defined as infection occurring within 90 days of a 2 day or longer hospitalization; in a nursing home or long-term care residency; within 30 days of receiving intravenous antibacterial therapy, chemotherapy, or wound care or after a hospital or hemodialysis clinic visit; or in any patient in contact with a multidrug resistant pathogen.

The pneumonia severity index (PSI) stratifies patients into 5 categories, and groups I and II may be treated as outpatients, while groups IV and V should be admitted for treatment. CURB-65 is calculates a score on criteria that include: confusion (disorientation to person, place, or time), urea (BUN>20), respiratory rate ($\geq$ 30), low blood pressure (SBP < 90 or DBP $\geq$60), and age $\geq$ 65.

- *Nazarian DJ, et al. clinical Policy: critical issues in the management of adult patients presenting to the emergency department with community acquired pneumonia. Ann Emerg Med 2009; 54(5): 704-731. full text*

Amy Kaji

- *MD Calc - CURB- 65. http://www.mdcalc.com/curb-65-severity-score-community-acquired-pneumonia/*

- *MD Calc - PSI. http://www.mdcalc.com/psi-port-score-pneumonia-severity-index-adult-cap/*

#21

Are routine blood cultures indicated in patients admitted with community acquired pneumonia?

    A. Yes, all patients admitted with CAP should have blood cultures drawn.

    B. Blood cultures may be considered in high-risk patients admitted with CAP (severe disease, immunocompromised, significant comorbidities, or other risk factors for infection with resistant organisms).

    C. Both of the above

    D. Neither of the above

#21

Answer: B

The 2007 American Thoracic Society and Infectious Disease Society of America guidelines recommended pretreatment blood cultures for those patients hospitalized with the following conditions: cavitary infiltrates, leukopenia, active alcohol abuse, chronic severe liver disease, asplenia, positive test result for pneumococcal urinary antigen, pleural effusion, or those admitted to the ICU. Blood cultures are optional for those without the specifically listed conditions. Blood cultures are infrequently positive, and the results do not often lead to change in management.

- Nazarian DJ, et al. Clinical policy: critical issues in the management of adult patients presenting to the emergency department with community acquired pneumonia. Ann Emerg Med. 2009; 54: 704-731. full text

- Mandell L, et al. Infectious Diseases Society of America/American Thoracic Society consensus guidelines on the management of community-acquired pneumonia in adults. Clin Infect Dis. 2007 Mar 1;44 Suppl 2:S27-72. full text

#22

Regarding the evaluation and management of adult patients presenting to the ED with suspected pulmonary embolism, which of the following statements is TRUE?

A. While both objective criteria and gestalt clinical assessment can be used to risk stratify patients with suspected PE, there is sufficient evidence to support the use of objective criteria.

B. Objective criteria include the Geneva Score, the Wells Score, the Kline Rule, and the Pisa Model.

C. Both of the above

D. Neither of the above

#22

Answer: B

Both objective criteria and gestalt assessment appear to perform equally well for patients with suspected PE. There were no Level A recommendations for the question: do objective criteria provide improved risk stratification over gestalt clinical assessment in the evaluation of patients with possible PE? However, it was a class B recommendation that either could be used, since there was insufficient evidence to support the use of one method over another.

• *ACEP clinical policy; Critical issues in the evaluation and management of adult patients presenting to the emergency department with suspected pulmonary embolism. Ann Emerg Med. 2011; 57: 628-652. full text*

#23

The utility of the Pulmonary Embolism Rule Out Criteria (PERC) rule is greatest in which of the following patients suspected of a pulmonary embolism?

    A. High pretest probability

    B. Intermediate pretest probability

    C. Low pretest probability

    D. No Pretest Probability

#23

Answer: C

As a class B recommendation, in patients with a low pretest probability for suspected PE, consider using the PERC to exclude the diagnosis based on historical and physical examination alone. The PERC require the clinician to answer "No" to 8 questions. If a patients is low risk by gestalt impression and is PERC negative, the post-test probability of venous thromboembolism is <2%.

The PERC rule criteria are:

1. Age $\geq$ 50 yo
2. HR $\geq$ 100 bpm
3. O_2 Sat < 95% on room air?
4. Is there a present history of hemoptysis?
5. Is the patient taking exogenous estrogen?
6. Does the patient have a prior diagnosis of venous thromboembolism (VTE)?
7. Has the patient had recent surgery or trauma? (Requiring endotracheal intubation or hospitalization in the previous 4 weeks.)
8. Does the patient have unilateral leg swelling? (Visual observation of asymmetry of the calves.)

The rule estimates the risk of PE at < 2%.

- *ACEP clinical policy: Critical issues in the evaluation and management of adult patients presenting to the emergency department with suspected pulmonary embolism. Ann Emerg Med. 2011 Jun; 57(6):628-652.e75. full text*

#24

The utility of a quantitative D-dimer test is greatest in which of the following patients suspected of a pulmonary embolism?

    A. Patients with a low pre-test probability

    B. Patients with an intermediate pre-test probability

    C. Patients with a high pre-test probability

#24

Answer: A

Despite consensus guidelines that recommend using D-dimer testing on patients with intermediate pretest probability for PE, strong evidence supporting this approach is lacking. Thus, D-dimer testing is indicated in low pre-test probability patients. Further research is necessary to determine the safety of d-dimer testing in intermediate risk populations.

- ACEP clinical policy: Critical issues in the evaluation and management of adult patients presenting to the emergency department with suspected pulmonary embolism. Ann Emerg Med. 2011 Jun; 57(6):628-652.e75. full text

#25

In which of the following patients can a negative CT pulmonary angiogram exclude the diagnosis of PE?

A. A patient with low pretest probability who had additional diagnostic testing performed because of a positive D-dimer

B. A patient with an intermediate pretest probability with a negative d-dimer

C. Both of the above

Amy Kaji

#25

Answer: C

If a patient is intermediate pretest probability, then additional diagnostic testing should be considered, such as a d-dimer, lower extremity imaging, VQ scanning, or traditional pulmonary angiogram prior to exclusion of venous thromboembolism (VTE). A negative highly sensitive quantitative d-dimer result in combination with a negative multidetector CT pulmonary angiogram result theoretically provides a posttest probability of VTE of less than 1%. The sensitivity of helical CTA for PE rule-out is estimated at 97%.

- *ACEP clinical policy: Critical issues in the evaluation and management of adult patients presenting to the emergency department with suspected pulmonary embolism. Ann Emerg Med. 2011 Jun; 57(6):628-652.e75. full text*

•Schoepf J, et al. Spiral Computed Tomography for Acute Pulmonary Embolism. Circulation. 2004; 109: 2160-2167. full text

#26

When would venous ultrasound be indicated as the initial imaging modality for evaluating a patient with symptoms consistent with pulmonary embolism (PE)?

A. Patients with obvious signs of DVT for whom venous ultrasound is readily available

B. Patients with borderline renal insufficiency

C. Patients with CT contrast agent allergy

D. Pregnant patient

E. All of the above

#26

Answer: E

This is a level B recommendation. A positive ultrasound in a patient with symptoms consistent with PE can be considered evidence for diagnosis of VTE and may preclude the need for additional diagnostic testing. Examples of situations in which venous ultrasound may be considered as initial imaging may include patients with obvious signs of DVT for whom ultrasound is readily available, and patients with relative contraindication for CT scan.

- *ACEP clinical policy: Critical issues in the evaluation and management of adult patients presenting to the emergency department with suspected pulmonary embolism. Ann Emerg Med. 2011 Jun; 57(6):628-652.e75. full text*

#27

Which of the following are indications to administer a thrombolytic therapy in patients with PE?

- A. Hemodynamically unstable patient with confirmed PE for whom the benefits of treatment outweigh the risks of life-threatening bleeding complications

- B. Hemodynamically stable patient with confirmed PE for whom the thrombus appears to be greater than 5 cm

- C. Both of the above

- D. Neither of the above

#27

Answer: A

The ACEP Clinical policy concludes that there is insufficient evidence to make any recommendations regarding use of thrombolytics in any subgroup of hemodynamically stable patients. Thrombolytics have been demonstrated to result in faster improvements in right ventricular function and pulmonary perfusion, as well as decreased pulmonary hypertension but these benefits have not translated to improvements in mortality. There are also significant bleeding risks associated with thrombolytic therapy.

A level C recommendation was given to consider thrombolytic therapy in hemodynamically unstable patients with a high clinical suspicion of PE for whom the diagnosis of PE cannot be confirmed in a timely manner.

For intermediate-risk PE: thrombolysis was associated with lower mortality (OR, 0.48; 95% CI, 0.25-0.92) but more major bleeding events (OR, 3.19; 95% CI, 2.07-4.92).

• ACEP clinical policy: Critical issues in the evaluation and management of adult patients presenting to the emergency department with suspected pulmonary embolism. Ann Emerg Med. 2011 Jun; 57(6):628-652.e75. full text

• Chatterjee S, et al. Thrombolysis for Pulmonary Embolism and Risk of All-Cause Mortality, Major Bleeding, and Intracranial Hemorrhage. JAMA. 2014. 311(23):2414-21. full text

#28

You are seeing a patient with a traumatic hemothorax. A chest tube is placed with 200cc of blood output. Indications for thoracotomy include which of the following?

A. Initial output of > 20 ml/kg of blood

B. Persistent bleeding at a rate of > 1 ml/kg/hr

C. Both of the above

D. Neither of the above

#28

Answer: A

Indications for thoracotomy after chest tube include initial tube drainage of 1500 ml or > 20 ml/kg of blood, and persistent bleeding at a rate of 200 ml or > 7 ml/kg/hr for three hours.

- *Rosen's Emergency Medicine - Concepts and Clinical Practice. 8th edition. 2013. Chapter 45: Thoracic Trauma. 441.*

#29

You are seeing a patient who presents with chest pain and shortness of breath. The chest X-ray demonstrates a right sided pleural effusion. TRUE statements about pleural effusions include which of the following?

(Choose three answers.)

A. In the absence of a bloody tap, bloody fluid suggests trauma, neoplasm, or pulmonary infarction.

B. If the hematocrit of the pleural fluid is more than 1% of the peripheral blood, the effusion is a hemothorax.

C. Post-expansion pulmonary edema is rare except when there are large volumes (>1500 ml) are drained in one session.

D. If this patient has congestive heart failure, diuretic therapy should be initiated.

E. Light's criteria for differentiating exudates from transudates requires measuring WBC in the pleural fluid and comparing it to the serum level.

#29

Answer: A, C, and D

Light's criteria include comparison of pleural fluid protein and pleural fluid lactate dehydrogenase level (LDH) to serum levels to differentiate an exudate from a transudate.

In evaluating a possible hemothorax, if the hematocrit of the pleural fluid is greater than 10% that of the peripheral blood, the effusion is a hemothorax.

For patients with CHF, pleural effusions generally respond well to diuretics.

After thoracentesis, transient hypoxia caused by ventilation-perfusion mismatch often occurs. Unilateral, post expansion pulmonary edema is rare except when large volumes are drained in one session (> 1500 ml).

• *Rosen's Emergency Medicine - Concepts and Clinical Practice. 8th edition. 2013. Chapter 77: Pleural Diseases. 992-996.*

#30

Which of the following statements is correct with respect to primary spontaneous pneumothorax and secondary spontaneous pneumothorax?

(Choose two answers.)

A. In most cases of secondary spontaneous pneumothorax, tube thoracostomy should be considered because less invasive approaches are associated with lower rates of success.

B. Suction should be applied for all patients after tube thoracostomy since it accelerates lung reexpansion.

C. For healthy young patients with a small (<20%) primary spontaneous pneumothorax, observation alone (with administration of 100% oxygen is an appropriate treatment option.

D. None of the above

E. All of the above

#30

Answer: A and C

Aspiration for spontaneous pneumothoraces that are larger than 20% can be performed with an IV catheter. If there is no recurrence of the pneumothorax after 6 hours, the patient can be discharged with close follow-up. Routine application of suction after tube thoracostomy is no longer recommended and does not accelerate lung reexpansion. Observation with oxygen therapy is also an option for patients with small pneumothoraces.

- *Rosen's Emergency Medicine - Concepts and Clinical Practice. 8th edition. 2013. Chapter 77: Pleural Diseases. 988-992.*

#31

True or False: Routine blood cultures are indicated in patients admitted for community acquired pneumonia (CAP).

    A. True

    B. False

#31

Answer: B

False, blood cultures should be considered in higher-risk patients admitted with CAP (severe disease, immunocompromised, significant comorbidities, or other risk factors for infection with resistant organisms. Blood culture results may be misleading and may cause unintended consequences, as false positives are common. Moreover, there are few data about blood culture performance in CAP patients and association with outcomes such as mortality, time to clinical stability, and length of stay. Antibiotic therapy is rarely changed based on blood culture results (0-5%).

• LLSA 2012: Nazarian DJ, et al. Clinical policy: critical issues in the management of adult patients presenting to the ED with Community Acquired Pneumonia. Ann Emerg Med. 2009; 704-731. full text

#32

The mechanisms that cause hypoxemia can be divided into those that increase $P(A-a)O_2$ and those where $P(A-a)O_2$ is preserved. Which of the following etiologies of hypoxemia increase the gradient?

(Choose two answers.)

    A. Hypoventilation

    B. Low inspired oxygen

    C. Right to left shunt

    D. Ventilation-perfusion inequality

    E. Diffusion impairment

#32

Answer: C and D

In diffusion impairment, the gradient is normal at rest but may be elevated during exercise. Impaired diffusion may occur when there is an increase in the thickness of the physical separation between alveolar gas and pulmonary capillary blood and a shortened pulmonary transit time.

The key clinical feature of a right to left shunt is that the accompanying hypoxemia does not correct with administration of supplemental oxygen. This is because the shunted blood is not exposed to the supplemental oxygen, and this lowers the overall arterial PO_2. V/Q mismatch is the most common cause of hypoxia. Normally, the alveolar ventilation is 4-6 L/min and pulmonary blood flow has a similar range. Thus, the normal range of ventilation-perfusion ratio for the whole lung is 0.8-1.2. Note that ventilation-perfusion must be matched at the individual alveolar-capillary level for gas exchange to be adequate.

Consider a hypothetical scenario where all pulmonary blood flow is directed to the right lung and all the ventilation is directed to the left lung. Although the whole lung V/Q ratio would be within the normal range, at the alveolar-capillary level, there would be NO gas exchange. There are regional variations in the V/Q ratio in the healthy upright lung, where the V/Q ratio decreases from the top to the bottom of the upright lung, and this normal pattern accounts for approximately 2/3 of the normal gradient seen in healthy individuals.

• Harris EA, et al. The normal alveolar-arterial oxygen tension gradient in man. Clin Sci Mol Med. 1974 Jan; 46(1): 89-104.

#33

True or False: In adults patients with community acquired pneumonia without severe sepsis, there is benefit in mortality and morbidity from the administration
of antibiotics within 4 hours.

A. True

B. False

#33

Answer: B

There is insufficient evidence to establish a benefit in mortality or morbidity from antibiotics administered in less than 4, 6, or 8 hours from ED arrival. In the most recent guidelines of CAP in adults, the Infectious Diseases Society of America and the American Thoracic Society agreed that there is limited data to support a specific time recommendation for the administration of antibiotics in ED patients with CAP. The recommendation states that for patients admitted through the ED, the first antibiotic dose should be administered while the patient is still in the ED.

• Nazarian DJ, et al. Clinical policy: critical issues in the management of adult patients presenting to the ED with CAP. Ann Emerg Med. 2009; 704-731. full text

• Mandell L, et al. Infectious Diseases Society of America/American Thoracic Society consensus guidelines on the management of community-acquired pneumonia in adults. Clin Infect Dis. 2007 Mar 1;44 Suppl 2:S27-72. full text

#34

What is the normal rate of resorption of a pneumothorax per day without any intervention?

A. About 5%

B. About 10%

C. About 1%

D. About 15%

E. About 20%

#34

Answer: C

The rate of resorption of a pneumothorax is approximately 1.25% per pneumothorax per 24 hours. By administering 100% humidified supplemental oxygen, the rate of resorption can be increased 6-fold (according to animal models). Note that recurrence of spontaneous pneumothorax is thought to occur in 25 to 54% of cases.

- Kelly AM, et al. Estimating the rate of re-expansion of spontaneous pneumothorax by a formula derived from computed tomography volumetry studies. Emerg Med J. Oct 2006; 23(10): 780–782. full text

RENAL AND VASCULAR

#1

A 75 year old male with diabetes and hypertension presents with pleuritic chest pain and hypoxia that is concerning for a pulmonary embolus. His medications include a thiazide and metformin. His creatinine is 1.9. Compression ultrasound is negative but you begin anti-coagulation for presumed PE and admit to the hospital-ist. The inpatient team plans on performing a CT with IV contrast. Prior to the CT scan, which of the following would NOT reduce the risk of contrast-induced nephr-opathy:

(Choose two answers.)

A. Withhold diuretics and NSAIDS for 24 hours be-fore and after the contrast administration.

B. Infusion of low osmolar agent (vs. high osmolar agent).

C. Withhold metformin for 48 hours before and after the contrast administration.

D. Intravenous fluid administration 1ml/kg per hour for 12 hours before and for 12 hours after the scan.

E. Single dose of N-acetylcysteine or bicarbonate administration.

#1
Answer: C and E

The use of bicarbonate or N-acetylcysteine is not routinely recommended in these patients because of the inconsistent results from clinical trials. While withholding metformin 48 hours before and after contrast administration decreases the rate of lactic acidosis associated with contrast-induced nephropathy, it does not decrease the rate of contrast-induced nephropathy. All of the other measures have been demonstrated to be helpful in reducing the risk of contrast-induced nephropathy.

- *LLSA 2008: Barrett BJ, et al. Preventing nephropathy induced by contrast medium. N Engl J Med. 2006 Jan 26; 354(4): 379-86.*

#2

Which of the following are complications of dialysis vascular access grafts?

A. Patients with borderline cardiac reserve and an excessive flow rate through their shunt may exhibit signs and symptoms of congestive heart failure.

B. An arterial steal syndrome with distal ischemia may occur in patients with shunts when the blood flows from the artery into the low-resistance vein with less arterial blood available distal to the site of the shunt.

C. Venous hypertension may also result from high pressure arterial flow into the low pressure venous system with resulting swelling of the distal tissue and eventual skin induration.

D. Neurovascular problems associated with vascular access include pain, weakness, muscular atrophy, and paresthesias.

E. All of the above

#2

Answer: E

All of the following complications can occur. Shunt repair may be necessary if the steal syndrome and venous hypertension cause clinical symptoms. These hemodynamic and neurovascular complications are more problematic with fistulas but can also occur with prosthetic grafts.

- *Roberts and Hedges' Clinical Procedures in Emergency Medicine. 6th edition. 2013. Chapter 24: Indwelling Vascular Devices: Emergency Access and Management. 444-453.*

#3

Which of the following is the most common cause of acute interstitial nephritis (AIN)?

    A. Viral infection

    B. Bacterial infection

    C. Immune-mediated disease

    D. Parasitic infection

    E. Drug hypersensitivity

#3

Answer: E

The most common cause of AIN is drug hypersensitivity. Commonly implicated drugs are beta-lactam antibiotics, sulfonamides, and NSAIDS. Presenting symptoms can include nonspecific findings such are arthralgia, rash, and eosinophiluria. Initially, in the ED, it is difficult to distinguish AIN from other causes of renal failure.

- *Rosen's Emergency Medicine - Concepts and Clinical Practice. 8th edition. 2013. Chapter 97: Renal Failure: 1293.*

#4

Which of the following would NOT be consistent with a pre-renal etiology for renal failure, and more consistent with acute tubular necrosis?

    A. BUN/Cr > 20:1

    B. Urine osmolarity < 350 mOsm/kg

    C. Urine Na < 20 mEq/L

    D. Urine specific gravity > 1.020

    E. Fractional excretion Na < 1%

#4

Answer: B

In pre-renal azotemia, the urine osmolarity would be expected to be high (greater than 500), but in ATN, it would be expected to be < 350 mOsm/kg. All of the other values are consistent with a pre-renal cause of acute renal failure. Additionally, the urinalysis in pre-renal failure would be expected to be either normal or demonstrate only hyaline casts.

- *Rosen's Emergency Medicine - Concepts and Clinical Practice. 8th edition. 2013. Chapter 97: Renal Failure. 1292.*

Amy Kaji

#5

You are seeing a nine year old with what appears to have nephrotic syndrome. All of the following are potential complications of nephrotic proteinuria EXCEPT?

A. Coagulopathy/bleeding

B. Infection

C. Thrombosis

D. Anasarca

E. Hypovolemia

Amy Kaji

#5

You are seeing a nine year old with what appears to have nephrotic syndrome. All of the following are potential complications of nephrotic proteinuria EXCEPT?

A. Coagulopathy/bleeding

B. Infection

C. Thrombosis

D. Anasarca

E. Hypovolemia

#5

Answer: A

Children with nephrotic syndrome have decreased humoral immunity leading to increased bacterial infections. The presence of ascites increases the incidence of spontaneous bacterial peritonitis. The decrease in oncotic pressure can leads to anasarca, causing pulmonary edema, effusions, and respiratory distress. There is also an increased risk of thrombosis but not bleeding. Hypovolemia can also occur, and in severe cases, progress to shock.

- *Rosen's Emergency Medicine - Concepts and Clinical Practice. 8th edition. 2013. Chapter 97: Renal Failure. 1294.*

Amy Kaji

#6

Loss of the vascular access is a major problem in hemo-dialysis, most cases being due to thrombosis of the access. In addition, other complications that may result from AV-graft or fistula placement include which of the following?

    A. High output congestive heart failure

    B. Seroma formation

    C. Ischemia distal to the fistula or graft

    D. Infection

    E. Pseudo-aneurysm

    F. All of the above

#6

Answer: F

Vascular access-related heart failure is rare, but after placement of all types of access, preexisting left ventricular hypertrophy can increase. The rate of heart failure is the same among access types. Weeping syndrome can occur when ultrafiltration of plasma across a graft, forms a pocket of fluid around the graft site. Seromas occur around graft sites where the pressure gradient is highest and develop slowly after months of graft implantation. Grafts, catheters, and fistulas are all at risk for infection due to repeat access. Staphylococcus aureus and, less commonly, Staphylococcus epidermidis are the predominant pathogens causing bacteremia.

Placement of an AV access can result in distal hypoperfusion of the extremity in patients with severe peripheral vascular disease due to shunting ("steal") of arterial blood flow into the fistula. Symptomatic steal occurs when there is a failure of adequate collateral flow and/or excessive fistula blood flow.

Aneurysms and pseudo-aneurysms are relatively infrequent complications of vascular access that usually result from repeated cannulation in the same area of the fistula. These problems can be avoided by rotation of needle insertion sites. Pseudo-aneurysms are a particular problem with poly-tetra-flourethylene (PTFE) grafts, occurring as the graft material deteriorates after prolonged use.

- *Roberts and Hedges' Clinical Procedures in Emergency Medicine. 6th edition. 2013. Chapter 24: Indwelling Vascular Devices: Emergency Access and Management. 440-453.*

#7

Regarding the diagnosis and management of post-streptococcal glomerulonephritis, which of the following is TRUE?

(Choose two answers.)

    A. Patients should be treated with 2-4 weeks of IV antibiotics.

    B. Most patients recover, particularly children.

    C. All patients present with hematuria, edema, and hypertension.

    D. The risk is greatest in those aged 20-40 yo.

    E. It is the most common cause of glomerulonephritis, worldwide.

#7
Answer: B and E

Poststreptococcal glomerulonephritis (PSGN) is the most common cause of acute nephritis worldwide. The risk of PSGN is greatest in children between 5 and 12 years of age, and older adults greater than 60 years of age. Beta-hemolytic streptococcus (GAS) causes a post infectious immune complex deposition. Clinical presentation varies and can range from mild edema and hypertension to gross hematuria, and renal failure.

Laboratory findings include an abnormal urinalysis (dysmorphic red blood cells, varying degrees of proteinuria, red blood cell casts, and pyuria), positive serology for antibodies to streptococcal antigens, and hypocomplementemia. PSGN is typically diagnosed based upon the findings of acute nephritis and demonstration of a recent GAS infection. Treatment is supportive and focused maintaining euvolemia, managing electrolytes and monitoring renal function. Recovery usually occurs in two weeks, but renal insufficiency can persist in severe cases.

• Rodríguez-Iturbe B, Batsford S. Pathogenesis of poststreptococcal glomerulonephritis a century after Clemens von Pirquet. Kidney Int. 2007 Jun; 71(11): 1094-104. full text

#8

Regarding rhabdomyolysis, which of the following statements is TRUE?

A. Myoglobin does not appear to be nephrotoxic in the renal tubules unless the urine is acidic.

B. The defined threshold value of serum creatine kinase above which renal damage always occurs has been defined as 5,000 IU/L.

C. Measurement of serum myoglobin is the most sensitive test for rhabdomyolysis.

D. Hypercalcemia is a common complication in the initial phases of rhabdomyolysis.

E. The fractional excretion of sodium is usually greater than 5%.

#8

Answer: A

Myoglobin does not actually have a nephrotoxic effect on the renal tubular system, unless the urine is acidic. Patients will have dipstick positive for blood without evidence of RBCs along with pigmented granular casts and increased serum creatine kinase (CK). Acute kidney injury is unlikely with CK levels less than 15,000 IU/L, but the patient should receive aggressive fluid administration. Patient with multiple comorbidities are still at risk for kidney injury with CK values as low as 5000 IU/L.

Myoglobin has an unpredictable metabolism, and correlation with levels of creatine kinase is poor. Serum myoglobin is a poor marker for detection of rhabdomyolysis and should not be measured in lieu of the total CK level.

While most forms of tubular necrosis will have an elevated fractional excretion (FENa) of sodium, rhabdomyolysis often has a low FENa (<1%). It is hypothesized that during rhabdomyolysis, vascular and tubular occlusion occurs, rather than tubular necrosis.

Hypocalcemia is a common complication of rhabdomyolysis and usually results from calcium entering the damaged muscle cells and from the precipitation of calcium phosphate with calcification in necrotic muscle. Hypercalcemia often occurs during the resolution of rhabdomyolysis due to the mobilization of calcium that was sequestered in the damaged muscle.

- *Bosch X, Poch E, Grau JM. Rhabdomyolysis and acute kidney injury. 2009 Jul 2; 361(1): 62-72.*

#9

TRUE statements about rhabdomyolysis include which of the following?

(Choose two answers.)

A. The triad of muscle pain, weakness, and dark urine will be seen in the majority of symptoms.

B. The serum CK begins to rise from 2 to 12 hours and peaks within 24 to 72 hours.

C. Myoglobin results in the production of red to brown urine.

D. Because of the long half-life of myoglobin, it will remain elevated and is a sensitive marker.

E. Hypokalemia and hypophosphatemia may result.

#9

Answer: B and C

More than half of patients may not report muscular symptoms, and only an occasional few will complain of pain (so the triad does not occur in the majority of patients). Serum CK is usually at least 5 times upper limit of normal at presentation and a decline generally occurs within 3-5 days. CK has a serum half-life of 1.5 days, whereas myoglobin has a half-life of only 2-3 hours. This large difference in the rate of metabolism makes measurement of myoglobin to detect rhabdomyolysis a very insensitive test. Myoglobinuria is absent in 25-50% of patients and hyperkalemia and hyperphosphatemia result from the release of potassium and phosphorus from damaged muscle cells.

- *Bosch X, Poch E, Grau JM. Rhabdomyolysis and acute kidney injury. N Engl J Med. Jul 2 2009; 361(1):62-72.*

#10

Complications from rhabdomyolysis include which of the following?

    A. Acute kidney injury (AKI)

    B. Compartment syndrome

    C. Disseminated intravascular coagulation

    D. A and B only

    E. A, B, and C.

#10

Answer: E

AKI is a common complication of rhabdomyolysis, and the reported frequency ranges from 15-50%. Risk factors for AKI include higher levels of CK, dehydration, sepsis, and acidosis. Compartment syndrome may develop after fluid resuscitation, and can further precipitate rhabdomyolysis. Infrequently, rhabdomyolysis may be associated with DIC, due to the release of prothrombotic substances from the damaged muscles.

- *Rosen's Emergency Medicine - Concepts and Clinical Practice. 8th edition. 2013. Chapter 97: Rhabdomyolysis. 1667-1675.*

Amy Kaji

#11

Causes of rhabdomyolysis include which of the following?

    A. Immobilization due to coma

    B. Crush syndrome

    C. Low-voltage electrical injury

    D. Severe hypokalemia

    E. Colchicine use

    F. A, B, and C

    G. A, B, D, and E

574

#11

Answer: G

There are multiple causes of rhabdomyolysis, and these can be broadly divided into three categories:

Traumatic or Muscle Compression:

1. Crush syndrome
2. Prolonged immobilization

Nontraumatic Exertional:

1. Intense physical exertion
2. Hyperthermia
3. Metabolic myopathies

Nontraumatic Nonexertional:

1. Drugs and toxins
2. Infections
3. Electrolyte disorders
4. High voltage electrical injuries
5. Extensive burns

Elaborating on a few of the causes, hypokalemia alters skeletal muscle blood flow by decreasing the normal vasodilation induced by potassium release by muscles. Many drugs, including statins and colchicine, are direct myotoxins. Both bacterial and viral infections have been associated with rhabdomyolysis.

• *Rosen's Emergency Medicine - Concepts and Clinical Practice. 8th edition. 2013. Chapter 97: Rhabdomyolysis. 1667-1675.*

• *Boomershine KH. Colchicine-induced rhabdomyolysis. Ann Pharmacother. 2002 May; 36(5): 824-6.*

• *Mannix R, Tan ML, Wright R, Baskin M. Acute pediatric rhabdomyolysis: causes and rates of renal failure. Pediatrics. Nov 2006; 118(5): 2119-25.*

#12

The treatment for rhabdomyolysis includes:

A. Fluid resuscitation and repletion until plasma CK is less than 5000 IU/L.

B. Calcium repletion in patients who have hypocalcemia.

C. Loop diuretics such as furosemide.

D. Fluid resuscitation with albumin.

#12

Answer: A

Early and aggressive fluid resuscitation is the major preventive therapy, and fluids should be administered until the CK values fall to < 5000. The optimal fluid for the prevention of rhabdomyolysis-induced AKI is not known. Loop diuretics have not been shown to be effective in preventing rhabdomyolysis-induced AKI but may be given to patients who develop volume overload. Calcium supplementation should be given only for symptomatic hypocalcemia or severe hyperkalemia.

- *Ratcliffe PJ, et al. Rhabdomyolysis in elderly people after collapse. Br Med J (Clin Res Ed). 1984 Jun 23; 288(6434): 1877-8. full text*

#13

Regarding rhabdomyolysis, which of the following statements is TRUE?

A. Acute kidney injury associated with myoglobinuria is the most serious complication of both traumatic and nontraumatic rhabdomyolysis.

B. The outcome of rhabdomyolysis is usually good provided that there is no renal failure.

C. Not all cases of rhabdomyolysis are associated with myoglobinuria.

D. Myoglobin seems to have no marked nephrotoxic effect in the tubules unless the urine is acidic.

E. Renal vasoconstriction is a characteristic feature of rhabdomyolysis-induced acute kidney injury.

F. All of the above

#13
Answer: F

All of these statements are true. Acute kidney injury is a complication of severe rhabdomyolysis and the prognosis is worse if renal failure develops. Approximately 7 to 10% of all cases of acute kidney injury in the United States are a result of rhabdomyolysis. Since myoglobin is a dark red 17.8-kDa protein that is freely filtered by the glomerulus, it appears in the urine only when it exceeds the renal threshold of 0.5 to 1.5 mg of myoglobin/dL. Patients will report their urine appearing reddish-brown ("tea-colored") at levels that exceed 100 mg per deciliter, so not all cases of rhabdomyolysis are associated with myoglobinuria. Myoglobin is nephrotoxic when the urine is acidic.

- Bozch X, et al. Rhabdomyolysis and Acute Kidney Injury. N Engl J Med. 2009; 361: 62-72. full text

#14

Regarding the management of rhabdomyolysis, which of the following statements is TRUE?

A. The most important aspect of treatment is early, aggressive fluid repletion.

B. One disadvantage of alkalinization of fluids is that it can exacerbate the hypercalcemia that is associated with the recovery phase of rhabdomyolysis.

C. Sodium bicarbonate infusion is clearly superior to saline infusion.

D. There are several randomized, controlled trials that support the evidence-based use of mannitol.

E. Early hypocalcemia should be treated aggressively.

#14

Answer: A

Patients with rhabdomyolysis present hypovolemic, not due intrinsic renal injury, but rather due to damaged muscle. The calcium influx into necrotic muscle also leads to free water sequestration. The main step in managing the condition remains early, aggressive repletion of fluids. Patient will often require up to 10 liters of fluid per day.

Bywaters and Beall proposed the first treatment with sodium bicarbonate in order to alkalinize the urine. However, this technique leads to hypocalcemia in an already hypocalemic state. Controversy still exists regarding sodium bicarbonate vs. normal saline or neutral fluid resuscitation. If sodium bicarbonate is used, urine pH and serum bicarbonate, calcium, and potassium levels should be monitored. If the urine pH does not rise after 4 to 6 hours of treatment or if hypocalcemia develops, alkalinization should be discontinued and hydration should be continued with normal saline.

Immediate correction of hyperkalemia is important as it can progress rapidly. Hypocalcemia should not be treated unless a patient is symptomatic or severe hyperkalemia is present. No randomized, controlled trial has supported the evidence-based use of mannitol, and some clinical studies suggest no benefit.

- *Bozch X, et al. Rhabdomyolysis and Acute Kidney Injury. N Eng J Med. 2009; 361: 62-72. full text*

- *Bywaters EGL, Beall D. Crush injuries with impairment of renal function. Br Med J. 1:427-432, 1941. full text*

#15

Regarding rhabdomyolysis, which of the following is TRUE?

    A. Myoglobin is removed by conventional hemodialysis.

    B. Conventional hemodialysis is indicated if the myoglobin level is greater than 500. IU/L

    C. Both of the above are true.

    D. Neither of the above is true.

#15
Answer: D

When acute kidney injury is severe enough to produce refractory hyperkalemia, acidosis, or volume overload, renal-replacement therapy is indicated, principally with intermittent hemodialysis, which can correct electrolyte abnormalities rapidly and efficiently. Conventional hemodialysis does not remove myoglobin due to the large size of the protein. Plasmapheresis also has no effect on outcomes or on the myoglobin levels. Continuous venovenous hemofiltration or hemodiafiltration has shown some efficacy in removing myoglobin, if employed with super high-flux filters and high volumes of ultrafiltration. The current evidence for these advanced techniques stem from case reports, and the effect on outcomes is unknown. Until randomized studies are performed demonstrating a clear benefit, routine hemofiltration is not recommended.

- *Bozch X, et al. Rhabdomyolysis and Acute Kidney Injury. N Eng J Med. 2009; 361: 62-72.*

#16

Which of the following is a renal manifestation of hypercalcemia?

    A. Diabetes insipidus

    B. Nephrocalcinosis

    C. Nephrolithiasis

    D. Acute and chronic renal failure

    E. Distal renal tubular acidosis

    F. All of the above

#16

Answer: F

Renal manifestation of hypercalcemia are, nephrolithiasis, renal insufficiency, and polyuria.

Nephrogenic diabetes insipidus - Although the mechanism is incompletely understood, hypercalcemia impairs the concentrating ability of the loop of Henle creating a degree of nephrogenic diabetes insipidus. The same effect on the loop of Henle can occur with the collecting tubules.

Nephrolithiasis - Chronic hypercalciuria usually from sarcoidosis, primary hyperparathyroidism, or medications can lead to nephrolithiasis.

Renal tubular acidosis - Chronic hypercalcemia infrequently causes type 1 (distal) renal tubular acidosis

Renal insufficiency - The development of renal insufficiency in individuals with hypercalcemia is related to the degree and duration of hypercalcemia. Higher elevations in the serum calcium concentration (serum calcium values of 12 to 15 mg/dL [3 to 3.75 mmol/L]) can lead to a decrease in the glomerular filtration rate

Renal failure - Chronic hypercalcemia can cause tubular calcification and atrophy and potentially progress to nephrocalcinosis. This progression is more prevalent in patients with sarcoidosis.

- *Rosen's Emergency Medicine - Concepts and Clinical Practice. 8th edition. 2013. Chapter 125: Electrolyte Disorders. 1645.*

#17

Which of the following is a gastrointestinal clinical manifestation of hypercalcemia?

    A. Anorexia

    B. Constipation

    C. Pancreatitis

    D. Peptic ulcer disease

    E. Nausea and vomiting

    F. A, B, D, and E

    G. A, B, C, D, and E

#17
Answer: G

Gastrointestinal symptoms, such as constipation, anorexia, and nausea occur commonly. Hypercalcemia causes changes in smooth muscle tone, which produce these gastrointestinal effects. Pancreatitis may develop due to calcium depositions in the pancreatic duct and activation of trypsinogen. Peptic ulcer disease and hypercalcemia occurs in the setting of hyperparathyroidism and increased gastrin secretion (MEN1 and Zollinger Ellison Syndrome).

- *Rosen's Emergency Medicine - Concepts and Clinical Practice. 8th edition. 2013. Chapter 125: Electrolyte Disorders. 1645.*

#18

A 45-year-old-woman with no history of venous thromboembolism presents with a proximal deep-vein thrombosis of her calf, diagnosed by compression duplex ultrasound. Which of the following statements is FALSE about the management?

A. Low-molecular-weight heparin is appropriate as initial therapy for this patient.

B. Oral anticoagulation should generally be started on the first day of treatment.

C. Thrombolytic therapy should be considered for patients less than 60 years of age who have limb-threatening circulatory compromise.

D. Inferior vena cava filters should be inserted in patients with contraindications to anticoagulation and in those who require urgent surgery that precludes anticoagulation.

E. In-patient hospitalization is recommended for initial treatment for most patients with deep-vein thrombosis.

#18

Answer: E

For most patients with deep-vein thrombosis, such as the patient described in the vignette, low-molecular-weight heparin (LMWH) administered on an outpatient basis is appropriate as initial therapy along with beginning an oral anticoagulant such as warfarin. If patients or family members cannot administer LMWH injections, home care should be arranged.

- *LLSA 2006: Bates SM, et al. Treatment of deep vein thrombosis. N Engl J Med. 2004; 351: 268-277.*

#19

One of the complications associated with vascular grafts involves erosion into contiguous structures with fistulization. Which of the following is FALSE regarding an aortoenteric fistula (AEF)?

A. Most commonly, these occur between an aortic prosthetic graft and the distal duodenum.

B. Mechanical trauma, prosthetic graft or perigraft infection and pressure necrosis all contribute to fistulization.

C. The time frame for AEF development is narrow; fistulization only occurs within the first few days post-operatively.

D. Clinical presentation is commonly that of gastrointestinal bleeding with hematemesis, hematochezia, melena, or occult blood loss.

E. Patients may present with self-limited herald bleeding several hours to days before exsanguinating hemorrhage.

#19

Answer: C

The time-frame from AEF development is wide. Fistulization may occur several days to many years after the initial surgery. All of the other statements are true.

- *Tagowski M, et al. Aortoenteric fistula as a complication of open reconstruction and endovascular repair of abdominal aorta. Radiol Res Pract. 2014; 2014: 383159. full text*

RHEUMATOLOGY

#1

You are treating a patient with a long history of gout who presents with acute right great toe pain, typical of his gouty flares. He is noncompliant with his medications. All of the following would be reasonable treatment options in the ED, EXCEPT:

A. Nonsteroidal anti-inflammatory drugs

B. Intra-articular steroids, if infection has been ruled out

C. Colchicine

D. Systemic steroids, if infection has been ruled out.

E. Allopurinol and probenecid

#1

Answer: E

Serum urate lowering agents, such as allopurinol and probenecid are contraindicated in the setting of acute or resolving gout. The resultant changes in the serum urate may exacerbate or prolong an attack. Joint rest and cold applications provide symptomatic relief. Warm compresses exacerbate joint inflammation and should be avoided. Narcotic analgesics provide further relief.

. Keith MP, Gilliland WR: Updates in the management of gout. Am J Med. 2007 Mar; 120(3): 221-4.

#2

You are seeing a 26 year old male with monoarticular arthritis of his right knee and you are concerned about gonococcal arthritis. Regarding the synovial fluid analysis, which of the following is FALSE?

A. Normal synovial fluid contains WBCs < 200/mm^3.

B. Leukocyte counts < 2000/mm^3 are considered non inflammatory and occur in osteoarthritis.

C. Greater than 2,000 WBCs indicate an inflammatory processes, but in septic arthritis WBCs are typically 50,000/mm^3 to 150,000/mm^3.

D. Synovial fluid chemistries, including glucose, protein, LDH, and lactate are highly sensitive and specific for septic arthritis and should be ordered whenever you suspect septic arthritis.

E. Gram stain and culture should be performed on every diagnostic specimen, since the gram stain is positive in 80% of gram positive infections although the sensitivity is much lower for gram negative infections.

#2

Answer: D

Note that an elevated synovial fluid leukocyte is not specific for infection, since rheumatoid and crystal arthropathy may induce significant inflammatory responses. Still, all synovial fluid samples should be analyzed for total leukocyte count with differential, gram stain, culture, and light microscopy for crystals. Culture remains the single most informative test if fluid is limited. Synovial fluid chemistries including LDH, glucose, protein, and lactate provide little additional information, and may be misleading.

- *Rosen's Emergency Medicine - Concepts and Clinical Practice. 8th edition. 2013. Chapter 116: Arthritis. 1508.*

#3

Which of the following is NOT a typical initial presentation of systemic lupus erythematosus (SLE)?

A. Weight gain

B. Fatigue

C. Fever

D. Anemia

E. Malar rash

#3

Answer: A

The most typical initial complaints with SLE are fatigue and migratory arthralgias (polyarticular), but fever, anemia, anorexia, and a malar rash are other common presenting symptoms. Arthralgias are often temporary and more often affect interphalangeal and metacarpophalangeal joints, wrists and knees.

- *Rosen's Emergency Medicine - Concepts and Clinical Practice. 8th edition. 2013. Chapter 118: Arthritis. 1527-1529.*

#4

Systemic manifestations of scleroderma include all of the following EXCEPT:

A. Cardiomyopathy

B. Restrictive lung disease

C. Gastrointestinal dysmotility

D. Malignant hypertension

E. All of the above

Amy Kaji

#4

Answer: E

Scleroderma is characterized by thickening of the skin caused by accumulation of collagen, and injury to small vasculature. The collagen can cause conduction defects, cardiomyopathies and pulmonary hypertension. Patients with significant restrictive lung disease will have interstitial fibrosis often visible on chest X-ray. The collagen depositions can also cause gastrointestinal motility problems, nutrient malabsorption, and severe renal arteriolar necrosis, which may lead to malignant hypertension.

- *Gabrielli A, Avvedimento E, Krieg T. Scleroderma. N Engl J Med. 2009 May 7; 360(19): 1989-2003.*

600

#5

Regarding Takayasu Arteritis, which of the following statements is FALSE?

A. It usually affects young women.

B. Has a predilection for involvement of the peripheral arteries (distal vasculature).

C. Patients may present with nonspecific symptoms of fever, night sweats, fatigue, myalgias, and weakness.

D. Myocardial ischemia and cerebrovascular accident may occur months to years after initial presentation.

E. Although rare, it should be considered in any young female patient with a CVA, upper extremity ischemia, or cardiac ischemia.

#5

Answer: B

Takayasu arteritis has a predilection for involvement of the aortic arch and large vessels. Women are affected up to 10 times more often than men, with peak incidence in the 3rd decade of life. Initial presenting symptoms are very nonspecific. Transient ischemic attack and CVA are seen in up to 5-10% of patients and are more often experienced by patients with carotid or vertebral disease. Myocardial infarctions are also not uncommon. Patients often requiring stenting of stenotic and dilated lesions of large- and medium-sized vasculature as well as anti-platelet therapy.

• *Rosen's Emergency Medicine - Concepts and Clinical Practice. 8th edition. 2013. Chapter 118: Systemic Lupus Erythematosus and the Vasculitides. 1535.*

#6

Regarding acute gouty arthritis, which of the following is FALSE?

A. NSAIDs are first-line therapy.

B. If the patient cannot tolerate NSAIDS, then intravenous colchicine is the next best agent for treatment.

C. Acute gout is an intensely painful inflammatory arthritis that typically involves a single joint, but can affect multiple joints.

D. Without therapy, acute gouty arthritis usually resolves within a few days to several weeks. However, symptoms improve more quickly with administration anti-inflammatory drugs.

E. Symptom resolution is more prompt and complete with early initiation of therapy.

#6

Answer: B

A number of drugs have been used for the treatment of acute gout. Although randomized trial data is surprisingly limited the following are effective:

- Nonsteroidal anti-inflammatory drugs
- Colchicine
- Intra-articular or systemic steroids
- Interleukin 1 beta inhibition (investigational).

There are no high-quality randomized, placebo-controlled trials of nonsteroidal anti-inflammatory drugs (NSAIDs) for acute gouty arthritis even though they are first line therapy and very little high quality evidence of colchicine. Regardless of therapy, patients will have decrease in pain over several days. Patients should also be instructed on the possible gastrointestinal irritation from NSAIDs and should avoid excessive intake. Colchicine can also cause gastrointestinal upset and diarrhea.

Oral colchicine can be effective for the treatment of acute gouty arthritis, particularly when administered early after the onset of symptoms. Intravenous colchicine has potentially serious adverse effects and since 2008 is not longer being distributed in the United States. IV colchicine was associated with bone marrow suppression, hepatic necrosis, acute renal failure, disseminated intravascular coagulation, seizures, and death. Significant tissue sclerosis can occur in the event of colchicine extravasation.

A safe, oral regimen for colchicine that is tolerated is 1.2mg followed 1 hour later by 0.6 mg for a total of 1.8mg daily.

- *Terkeltaub RA, et al. High versus low dosing of oral colchicine for early acute gout flare: Twenty-four-hour outcome of the first multi-*

center, randomized, double-blind, placebo-controlled, parallel-group, dose-comparison colchicine study. Arthritis Rheum. 2010 Apr; 62(4): 1060-8.

- Keith MP, Gilliland WR. Updates in the management of gout. Am J Med. 2007 Mar; 120(3): 221-4.

#7

You are seeing a patient in whom you suspect gouty arthritis. True statements about gout and pseudogout include all of the following, EXCEPT:

    A. Gout and pseudogout are the 2 most common crystal-induced arthropathies.

    B. Treatment of the acute phase of pseudogout is identical to that of gout.

    C. Similar to gout, there are effective medications to treat and prevent pseudogout.

    D. Other than the great toe, the most common sites of gouty arthritis are the ankle, wrist, and knee. The most common sites of pseudogout arthritis are the knee, wrist, and shoulder.

    E. Crystal-induced arthritis is most commonly monoarticular; however, polyarticular acute flares can also occur.

#7

Answer: C

Pseudogout is inflammation caused by calcium pyrophosphate (CPP) crystals and is sometimes referred to as calcium pyrophosphate disease (CPPD). Kohn et al discovered pseudogout as a disease process in 1962. The treatment of pseudogout is focused on pain relief with NSAIDs, but unlike gout, there are no targeted therapies to treat chronic symptoms or prevent recurrences.

- *Rosen's Emergency Medicine - Concepts and Clinical Practice. 8th edition. 2013. Chapter 116: Arthritis. 1509-1510.*

- *Kohn NN, et al. The significance of calcium phosphate crystals in the synovial fluid of arthritic patients: the "pseudogout syndrome. II. Identification of crystals. Ann Intern Med. 1962 May; 56: 738-45.*

#8

**Unless it is frankly bloody, traumatic non-septic ole-
cranon bursitis usually has a leukocyte count less than
_____, whereas septic bursal fluid has greater than
_____ white blood cells/mL.**

A. 100, 1000

B. 200, 1100

C. 1000, 10,0000

D. 50, 500

E. None of the above.

#8

Answer C

In evaluating a patient with suspected bursitis, similar to arthritis, it is important to differentiate a septic from an inflammatory process. Although this can often be accomplished based on history and physical, aspiration of the bursa can be performed and sent for crystals, cell count, gram's stain and culture. Unless it is frankly bloody, traumatic non-septic olecranon bursitis usually has a leukocyte count of less than 1000/mL whereas septic bursal fluid usually has greater than 10,000/mL WBCs.

- *Rosen's Emergency Medicine - Concepts and Clinical Practice. 8th edition. 2013. Chapter 117: Tendinopathy and Bursitis. 1524.*

#9

Regarding septic bursitis, which of the following statements is FALSE?

A. Olecranon and prepatellar bursitis is usually from direct inoculation related to trauma while trochanteric or iliopsoas result from hematogenous spread of infection.

B. Similar to septic arthritis, the cell counts from the bursa from septic bursitis are typically diagnostic with WBCs of > 50,000/mL .

C. Staph aureus is the causative organism in more than 80% of cases.

D. Imaging may be necessary to assess for the presence of deep bursal effusions.

E. Optimal duration of treatment is unknown, but typically for 2 weeks.

#9

Answer: B

Superficial bursae (olecranon and pre-patellar) are pre-disposed to direct inoculation related to trauma while septic deep bursitis (trochanteric or iliopsoas), is typically due to hematogenous spread. Pain and restricted joint motion may indicate septic bursitis. The vast majority of cases are caused by staphylococcus aureus, with streptococci species causing the remainder. The diagnosis of septic bursitis is mainly a clinical diagnosis with bursal fluid culture confirming the diagnosis. Imaging may be considered in the setting of trauma.

The range of septic bursal fluid WBCs is wide with no clear absolute threshold, similar to septic arthritis. The bursal glucose to serum glucose ratio may be the best test with values < 50% highly suggestive of infection. Accepted cutoffs for bursal WBCs in septic bursitis are 1000-5000/mL with > 5000/mL highly suggestive. These values are significantly lower than in septic arthritis.

Treatment of septic bursitis requires appropriate antibiotics directed against Staphylococcus and Streptococcus species and often paired with repeated drainage of the bursa.

- *Rosen's Emergency Medicine - Concepts and Clinical Practice. 8th edition. 2013. Chapter 117: Tendinopathy and Bursitis. 1524-1525.*

TOXICOLOGY

#1

Regarding carbon monoxide exposure, which of the following statements is FALSE?

    A. For the vast majority of patients, hyperbaric oxygen is administered as a lifesaving therapy.

    B. The half life of carboxyhemoglobin (COHb) is inversely related to the partial pressure of oxygen PO_2.

    C. Hyperbaric oxygen reduces the half life of COHb less than 40 minutes.

    D. Risk factors that predict the development of delayed neurologic sequelae from carbon monoxide include age and loss of consciousness.

    E. Special consideration should be given to the pregnant patient who is exposed to carbon monoxide, since fetal hemoglobin has a higher affinity for carbon monoxide.

Amy Kaji

#1

Answer: A

The half life of COHb can be reduced from approximately 5 hours on room air to 1 hour by providing supplemental 100% O_2. Few patients can be treated rapidly enough with hyperbaric oxygen such that it would be lifesaving. Under hyperbaric conditions, a sufficient O_2 can be achieved to sustain life in the absence of an adequately functioning hemoglobin, but this is relevant in situations in which the COHb is extremely elevated (e.g., > 50%). Thus, the primary indication for hyperbaric oxygen is to prevent delayed neurologic sequelae. Risk factors for delayed neurologic sequelae also include an abnormal cerebellar exam and COHb greater than 25%. A simple rule-of-thumb for COHb half-lives is 0.5 hrs on hyperbaric oxygen, 1.5 hrs on 100% normobaric oxygen, and 4.5 hrs on room air.

- Rosen's Emergency Medicine - Concepts and Clinical Practice. 8th edition. 2013. Chapter 159: Inhaled Toxins. 2440-2443.

- Goldfrank's Toxicologic Emergencies. 10th edition. 2014. Chapter 105: Carbon Monoxide.

- Weaver LK, et al. Hyperbaric oxygen for acute carbon monoxide poisoning. N Engl J Med. 2002; 347(14):1057-67.

#2

Regarding gamma-hydroxybutyrate (GHB), which of the following statements is FALSE?

A. Behavioral changes are most common with GHB intoxication and range from aggression and delirium to coma.

B. A distinctive feature of GHB intoxication is altered mental status with rapid and complete resolution.

C. Prolonged coma for many days is a common presentation.

D. GHB is not usually detected on most urine toxicology screens.

E. Withdrawal from GHB can manifest mildly with anxiety and tremor, but it can progress to a severe syndrome characterized by delirium and autonomic instability.

#2

Answer: C

GHB does not cause prolonged coma. Instead, it results in rapid resolution of symptoms unless there are concomitant co-ingestions. Patients usually awaken within 3-4 hours but may require respiratory support depending on the dose ingested. Alcohol is often ingested along with GHB and can prolong altered mental status but almost all patients recover within 6 hours. Cardiac effects and refractory seizures are uncommon, and either of these findings suggest the presence of another agent. Patients may present with significant vomiting and require intubation for airway protection. Treatment for GHB withdrawal is support with benzodiazepines, and if refractory, barbiturates and propofol should be used for severe GHB withdrawal.

• *Rosen's Emergency Medicine - Concepts and Clinical Practice. 8th edition. 2013. Chapter 165: Sedative Hypnotics. 2082-2083.*

• *Goldfrank's Toxicologic Emergencies. 10th edition. 2014. Chapter 83: Gamma-Hydroxybutyric Acid.*

#3

The most common early feature and symptom of quinine overdose is:

A. Cinchonism

B. Cardiac toxicity

C. Visual disturbances

D. Hypoglycemia

E. Thrombocytopenia

#3

Answer: A

While all of the above complications can occur with quinine overdose, cinchonism is the most common early feature, occurring in about 75% of patients. It usually occurs within 4 hours of ingestion but may appear as early as 2 hours and as late as 8 to 12 hours after ingestion. Cinchonism can be seen with acute and chronic poisoning and is characterized by tinnitus, hearing loss, nausea, vomiting, vertigo, ataxia, lethargy, and hypotension.

• *Goldfrank's Toxicologic Emergencies. 10th edition. 2014. Chapter 59: Antimalarials. 803-804.*

#4

Regarding isoniazid overdose, which of the following statements is FALSE?

A. Multiple seizures over a short time period are the hallmark of INH poisoning.

B. Seizures may be seen after acute overdoses of INH as low as 35 mg/kg in adults, and death has resulted after the ingestion of as little as 3 grams.

C. Phenytoin is the treatment of choice for refractory seizures.

D. Diazepam may be used as an adjunct to control seizures.

E. Severe metabolic acidosis may be seen.

#4

Answer: C

Pyridoxine (vitamin B6) is the antidote for INH overdose and should be given gram-for-gram for the total ingested amount of INH. When the dose of INH is unknown, 5 g of pyridoxine should be given empirically, and can be repeated after 20 minutes if there is no cessation of seizure activity. Benzodiazepines may be used as an adjunct to control seizures. Patients can also develop a concomitant lactic acidosis, due to seizures, which resolves after seizures abate and adequate fluid resuscitation is provided.

- Goldfrank's Toxicologic Emergencies. 10th edition. 2014. Chapter 58: Antituberculous Medications. 789-790.

#5

Regarding the use of atropine in the treatment of organophosphate insecticide poisoning, which of the following statements is FALSE?

A. Atropine should be titrated to endpoints, such as tachycardia and mydriasis.

B. Atropine may be repeated every 5 to 15 minutes, with consideration of an atropine infusion.

C. Atropine has no effect on nicotinic receptors and therefore will not reverse muscle weakness or sympathetic ganglionic effects.

D. Atropine acts by competitively blocking acetylcholine at muscarinic receptors, thereby reversing the excessive parasympathetic stimulation.

E. It is only partially effective in treating CNS symptoms and has a variable effect on seizures and altered mental status.

#5

Answer: A

Repeated doses of atropine may be needed to decrease bronchorrhea and oropharyngeal secretions. Atropine should be titrated to the drying of secretions and not to irrelevant endpoints such as mydriasis or tachycardia. Very often, tachycardia is a result of dyspnea and inadequate atropine dosing.

- *Rosen's Emergency Medicine - Concepts and Clinical Practice. 8th edition. 2013. Chapter 163: Pesticides. 2057-2060.*

#6

Regarding mushroom ingestion, which of the following statements is FALSE?

 A. Supportive care is the mainstay for management of any toxic mushroom ingestion.

 B. Most patients will not need therapy other than intravenous fluids and antiemetics.

 C. The most important historical piece of information is whether the mushroom was ingested with alcohol.

 D. Patients with hallucinations should be placed in a quiet, dark low stimulus environment.

 E. Benzodiazepines should be administered for seizures and severe agitation or hallucinations.

#6

Answer: C

Of greatest importance in the history is the time interval between ingestion of the mushroom and the onset of symptoms. Patients who present with GI symptoms that begin within 2 hours after ingestion, respond to IV fluids, and tolerate oral food and fluids, may be discharged unless there is a possibility of Amanita smithiana ingestion. Patients who develop symptoms 6 to 8 hours after ingestion should be admitted to the hospital. Consultation with regional poison control centers or a toxicologist is recommended.

- *Rosen's Emergency Medicine - Concepts and Clinical Practice. 8th edition. 2013. Chapter 164: Plants, Mushrooms, and Herbal Medications. 2074-2075.*

#7
Regarding ciguatera poisoning, which of the following statements is FALSE?

A. Ciguatera poisoning is endemic in the Australia, the Caribbean, and the South Pacific islands, with French Polynesia having the highest incidence.

B. It is due to the muscles of fish which contain large amounts of free histidine and become toxic when left unrefrigerated, allowing bacteria, particularly Proteus, to decarboxylate histidine to histamine.

C. Patients may have an intense burning sensation on exposure to cold.

D. Patients may have asthenia, paresthesias, joint pains, headaches, and describe a sensation of looseness of the teeth.

E. GI symptoms usually resolve by 24 to 48 hours and neurologic symptoms by 3 weeks.

#7

Answer: B

Ciguatera poisoning results from eating fish contaminated with toxins produced by dinoflagellates living in coral reef waters. The toxins are passed up the food chain from herbivores to their predators and eventually to humans. Ciguatoxin is a heat-stable, lipid soluble, tasteless and odorless toxin that is not destroyed by cooking or gastric acid.

Scombroid poisoning is associated with ingestion of fish whose muscles have large amounts of free histidine. The fish become toxic when left unrefrigerated and allow bacteria to decarboxylate the histidine to histamine.

- *Goldfrank's Toxicologic Emergencies. 10th edition. 2014. Chapter 44: Food Poisoning. 586-588.*

#8

Regarding cyanide toxicity, all of the following are true EXCEPT:

A. Common commercial uses of cyanide include synthetic fiber manufacturing, photographic industries and metalworking.

B. Hydrogen cyanide toxicity is due to its inhibition of tissue oxygen extraction from the blood.

C. Empiric therapy with the cyanide antidote kit (amyl nitrite, sodium nitrite, and sodium thiosulfate) or hydroxocobalamin should not be instituted until a diagnosis can be confirmed.

D. Oral cyanide ingestion may require prolonged therapy.

#8

Answer: C

Gaseous cyanide (often from fires or commercial exposures) is rapidly absorbed and inhibits oxidative metabolism by disrupting the electron transport chain. Tissue hypoxia occurs within seconds to minutes with profound effects on CNS and cardiovascular system due to the inability of the tissues to extract oxygen from the bloodstream. An increased anion gap metabolic acidosis and elevated serum lactate occur. Therapy should not be delayed in patients with suspected acute cyanide poisoning.

  • *Rosen's Emergency Medicine - Concepts and Clinical Practice. 8th edition. 2013. Chapter 159: Inhaled Toxins. 2039-2041.*

#9

A 14 year-old girl with a history of a "brain tumor" is brought in by EMS for a seizure at school; vitals and blood sugar in the field were normal. A school administrator accompanies the child and has limited information, other than she has been to the school nurse every day this week for headaches. Her emergency card from the school reveals that she is on carbamazepine (Tegretol). Her vital signs are normal, except for a HR of 120. She is stuporous and during your assessment has a generalized tonic-clonic seizure. You give 2 doses of 2 mg of Lorazepam IV, then give 20 mg/kg of Fosphenytoin over 5-10 minutes. She continues to seize, and as you are about to prepare for intubation, your point of care labs read:

pH 7.2; pCO2 50; Na 110; K 4.6; HCO3 14.

What is the next step in management of this patient?

A. Give Phenobarbital.

B. Give Keppra.

C. Give 20 mL/kg of NS IV and reassess.

D. Give 20 mL/kg NS IV while you prepare to give 4-6 mL/kg 3% saline.

#9

Answer: D

Although you have limited information about this patient, she has possible reasons to have syndrome of inappropriate antidiuretic hormone secretion (SIADH):

1. CNS neoplasm (which may just be her seizure focus and cause of headaches)
2. Carbamazepine

However, the fact that her seizure is not controlled with conventional therapy is suspicious. The confirmation that her serum sodium is dangerously low makes the diagnosis. This girl's serum sodium must be raised acutely to avoid ongoing neuronal damage. The rate of the symptoms (acute-seizure) should match the rate of correction (aggressive-hypertonic saline). (This is not the case in the patient who presents with weeks of symptoms, a normal exam, and a low Na+ on laboratory investigation.)

In this patient's case, NS is still hypertonic to the patient's serum sodium. It is reasonable to give while preparing the hypertonic 3% saline. The goal is to raise the patient's serum sodium by only a few mEq rapidly to increase her seizure threshold. The pediatric dose is 4-6 mL/kg 3% saline, half over 10 minutes and the other half over 50 minutes. The adult dose is based upon raising the serum sodium by 5 mEq/kg with 3% saline (in a 60 kg male, this is approximately 350cc of 3% saline); give 100 mL over 10 minutes and the remaining 250 mL over 50 minutes and repeat a chemistry panel.

This aggressive therapy violates the rule of correction of 1-2 mEq Na/hour, but does not violate the (more important) rule of correction of 10-12 mEq/Na/day in order to prevent central pontine myelinolysis.

- *Rosen's Emergency Medicine - Concepts and Clinical Practice. 2013. Chapter 125: Electrolyte Disorders. 1642-1645.*

#10

Regarding marijuana (THC), which of the following statements is FALSE?

A. Urinary metabolites of THC are detectable within 1 hour after smoking marijuana.

B. Positive urine tests may persist for three months after chronic marijuana use.

C. A positive urine test correlates with acute intoxication.

D. Inadvertent or passive exposure to marijuana can produce positive urine testing.

E. False positive urine screen results may be produced by non-steroidal analgesic medications, such as ibuprofen and naproxen.

#10
Answer: C

Adverse reactions to marijuana are rare, and no deaths have been solely attributed to marijuana. The most common adverse reaction is panic, paranoia, or acute psychosis. A positive urine test does not correlate with acute intoxication, since a single marijuana cigarette can be detected for 72 hours when a 100 ng/ml cutoff is used, and positive urine levels may persist for 3 months after chronic marijuana use. Nonsteroidal anti-inflammatory drugs have been reported to cause false positives on marijuana drug screens.

- *Rosen's Emergency Medicine - Concepts and Clinical Practice. 2013. Chapter 156: Hallucinogens. 2020-2022.*

- *Moeller KE, et al. Urine drug screening: practical guide for clinicians. Mayo Clin Proc. 2008 Jan;83(1):66-76. full text*

Amy Kaji

#11

Regarding the patient who may have concurrent toxicity from carbon monoxide and cyanide, which of the following is TRUE?

A. Smoke inhalation victims who present with coma and metabolic acidosis can have severe carbon monoxide poisoning, cyanide poisoning, or both.

B. Nitrite induced methemoglobinemia, which further reduces oxygen delivery, may be detrimental to patients with elevated COHb levels.

C. Sodium thiosulfate, administered alone, is shown to be beneficial and safe in dual cyanide - carbon monoxide poisonings.

D. If you can not exclude cyanide poisoning in a smoke inhalation victim with coma, hypotension, acidosis or cardiovascular collapse, then a standard dose of sodium thiosulfate (or hydroxocobalamin, if available) should be administered.

E. All of the above

#11

Answer: E

All of the above statements are true. If the COHb level is found to be low and the patient has persistent acidosis or hemodynamic instability, the complete cyanide antidote kit, including the nitrites, can be administered. Alternatively, if available, hydroxocobalamin can be administered with or without thiosulfate. Patients with high COHb levels undergoing therapy in a hyperbaric oxygen chamber can also receive nitrite therapy while pressurized, with little concern of decreasing the oxygen carrying capacity.

- Rosen's Emergency Medicine - Concepts and Clinical Practice. 8th edition. 2013. Chapter 159: Inhaled Toxins. 2042-2043.

- EMCrit - Cardiac Arrest after Smoke Inhalation with Lewis Nelson http://emcrit.org/podcasts/cardiac-arrest-after-smoke-inhalation/

#12

A patient with a history of bipolar disorder presents with lethargy, increased tremor, and dehydration. You suspect lithium toxicity. Which of the following statements is TRUE?

A. A high anion gap is typical in the patient who has chronic lithium toxicity.

B. Patients with lithium toxicity are classically volume overloaded.

C. Activated charcoal is of proven benefit in chronic lithium toxicity.

D. Diabetes insipidus may result from therapeutic use and toxic ingestions.

E. Hyperthyroidism may result from lithium toxicity.

#12

Answer: D

Lithium inhibits arginine vasopressin and impairs sodium and water conservation. Diabetes insipidus results from both therapeutic use and toxicity. The replacement of free water at rates of 1 L per hour is sometimes necessary, and patients are often volume depleted (not volume overloaded). Lithium has an antithyroid effect, and myxedema coma has been reported as a complication of toxicity (but not hyperthyroidism). A low anion gap (not a high anion gap) may suggest lithium toxicity. As with most elemental cations, activated charcoal is of little benefit, except in the case of coingestions. Although dialysis dramatically shortens the half-life, outcome studies have not demonstrated its benefit in chronic toxicity. However, dialysis should be used in the case of an acute overdose with decreased level of consciousness, seizures, renal failure and symptomatic patients with levels greater than 4 mEq/L. For chronic toxicity, dialysis may be helpful in symptomatic patients with levels greater than 2 mEq/L.

•   *Rosen's Emergency Medicine - Concepts and Clinical Practice. 8th edition. 2013. Chapter 160: Lithium. 2044-2046.*

#13

A patient presents with a acetaminophen overdose. You are about to use the Rumack-Matthew nomogram. In which type of ingestion can this nomogram guide you in diagnosis and treatment?

- A. Acute single ingestion with known time of ingestion.
- B. Repeated ingestions.
- C. Chronic ingestions.
- D. Unknown ingestion time period.
- E. All of the above are scenarios in which the nomogram can be used.

#13

Answer: A

The Rumack–Matthew nomogram was published in 1975 to estimate the likelihood of hepatic injury due to acetaminophen toxicity for patients with a single ingestion at a known time. The patient's plasma acetaminophen concentration and the time interval since ingestion are plotted and compared against the nomogram line. If the plotted point is above and to the right of the line then there is a risk of hepatic injury and n-acetylcysteine should be administered. If the point is below and to the left of the line, hepatic injury is unlikely. Timing of the nomogram starts at 4 hours. Patients with repeated supratherapeutic ingestions or with an unknown time of ingestion cannot be evaluated with the use of the Rumack–Matthew nomogram.

- *Heard KJ. Acetylcysteine for Acetaminophen poisoning. N Engl J Med. 2008 Jul 17; 359(3): 285-92. full text*

#14

You are seeing a glass-etcher who has an injury to his right hand after he believes that hydrofluoric acid spilled on it. He is complaining of severe pain. Which of the following is NOT appropriate for managing this patient?

A. Copious irrigation

B. Calcium gluconate gel

C. Systemic calcium administration

D. Succinylcholine injection into the wound

E. Cardiac monitoring

#14

Answer: D

Symptomatic hydrofluoric acid (HF) burns are treated with water irrigation and calcium. The fluoride ions form complexes with calcium due to their opposing charges. In severe toxicities, this can lead to hypocalcemia either locally at the wound site or systemically. To treat local hypocalcemia, 2.5% calcium gluconate gel can be applied for an hour. If it is difficult to apply the calcium to a hand wound, the gel can be placed in a surgical glove which is then placed on the hand. Topical calcium gluconate will also decrease the pain as the fluoride ions are bound to the topical calcium.

Patients with inhalation injuries should be treated with oxygen and nebulized calcium gluconate (4 ml of 2.5 to 5%). If a patient requires intubation, avoid succinylcholine due to the possibility of hyperkalemia.

HF burns can lead to systemic toxicity resulting in severe electrolyte abnormalities, particularly hypocalcemia and hyperkalemia. If systemic toxicity is suspected (due to QTc prolongation, cardiac arrhythmia, or obvious systemic illness), calcium should be administered intravenously. Calcium gluconate can be given as 1000 mg (10 mL of a 10% solution) infused slowly over two to three minutes; several repeat doses may be necessary if profound hypocalcemia is present. In cases of systemic toxicity, magnesium replacement (4 g IV over 20 minutes) is often required.

• *Rosen's Emergency Medicine - Concepts and Clinical Practice. 8th edition. 2013. Chapter 64: Chemical Injuries. 820-821.*

#15

What are the two earliest signs of phenytoin toxicity?

(Choose two answers.)

    A. Nausea and vomiting

    B. Rash

    C. Difficulty breathing

    D. Unsteady gait

    E. Horizontal nystagmus

#15
Answer: D and E

The earliest signs of phenytoin toxicity are horizontal nystagmus and unsteady gait. More severe toxicity results in slurred speech, along with a gradually worsening mental status lethargy, and altered mental status. Hyperreflexia is occasionally seen. There is no absolute correlation between drug level and clinical findings.

Although oral phenytoin does not cause cardiac complications, intravenous infusions of phenytoin or fosphenytoin can cause hypotension and bradyarrhythmias. With phenytoin, the hypotension is attributed to the effects of the diluent, propylene glycol.

- *Goldfrank's Toxicologic Emergencies. 10th edition. 2014. Chapter 48: Antiepileptics. 649-650.*

#16

You are seeing a patient who has a history of schizo-phrenia who states that she drank a few bottles of digoxin because some voices were telling her to do so. She says that she took the medications at 6am this morning. It is now 8am. When should the level of digoxin be checked?

A. Now

B. 9am

C. 10am

D. 11am

E. 12pm

#16

Answer: E

Plasma digoxin levels should be measured at least 6 hours after the last dose, since this is the time required for steady state. Measurements made earlier than steady state can present significantly higher.

The plasma digoxin concentration should be used only as a guide to appropriate therapeutic dosing and as an indicator of toxicity. Several factors (such as hypokalemia) can cause toxicity at levels less than 2 ng/mL (2.6 nmol/L). patients can also be asymptomatic with levels above 3 ng/mL (3.8 nmol/L)

Although the recommendation is to check a 6-8 hour digoxin level, a patient who has a level greater than 10-20 ng/mL obtained before the 6 hour mark will also likely demonstrate a toxic level at 6 hours.

- *Rosen's Emergency Medicine - Concepts and Clinical Practice. 8th edition. 2013. Chapter 152: Cardiovascular Drugs. 1982-1986.*

#17

Digoxin-specific Fab fragments are indicated in which of the following scenarios?

    A. Digoxin toxicity with hemodynamic instability

    B. Severe bradycardia

    C. Serum digoxin > 10 ng/ml

    D. Ingestion of greater than 10g of digoxin in an adult

    E. Ingestion of greater than 4g of digoxin in a child

    F. All of the above

#17

Answer: F

Digoxin-specific Fab fragments are indicated in the following settings:

1. Hemodynamic instability due to acute ingestion
2. Arrhythmias (atrial tachycardia with a 2:1 conduction, bidirectional ventricular tachycardia and atrial fibrillation with a slow ventricular response)
3. Severe bradycardia
4. A plasma potassium concentration above 5 mEq/L in the setting of acute overdose
5. Plasma digoxin concentration above 10 ng/mL (13 nmol/L)
6. Ingestion of > 10 mg of digoxin in adults or > 4 mg in children

Even if atropine corrects the bradycardia, digoxin-specific Fab fragments should be given to prevent a recurrent episode of bradycardia.

- *Rosen's Emergency Medicine - Concepts and Clinical Practice. 8th edition. 2013. Chapter 152: Cardiovascular Drugs. 1985.*

#18

You are seeing a patient in whom you suspect exposure to carbon monoxide. Indications for hyperbaric oxygen treatment include which of the following?

    A. Carboxyhemoglobin > 25%

    B. Age < 1 year of > 65

    C. Loss of consciousness

    D. Pregnancy by itself

    E. Metabolic alkalosis

#18

Answer: A and C

Hyperbaric oxygen therapy (HBO) involves exposing patients to 100% oxygen under supra-atmospheric conditions. Under hyperbaric conditions, the half life of carboxyhemoglobin decreases to 30 minutes. Contrast this with 90 minutes on 100% normobaric oxygen. The amount of oxygen dissolved in the blood also rises from approximately 0.3 to 6.0 mL per dL, which substantially increases the delivery of non-hemoglobin-bound oxygen to the peripheral tissues. Although HBO therapy has been criticized due to flawed randomized trials, the generally accepted recommendations for consideration of HBO treatment include:

1. Evidence of ongoing end-organ ischemia (eg, profound metabolic acidosis (pH <7.1), myocardial ischemia)

2. Loss of consciousness

3. Pregnant women with a COHb >15%, or evidence of fetal distress.

The goal of HBO therapy is to decrease long term neurologic impairment.

References:

- *Rosen's Emergency Medicine - Concepts and Clinical Practice. 8th edition. 2013. Chapter 159: Inhaled Toxins. 2440-2443.*

- *Goldfrank's Toxicologic Emergencies. 10th edition. 2014. Chapter 105: Carbon Monoxide.*

- *Weaver LK, et al. Hyperbaric oxygen for acute carbon monoxide poisoning. N Engl J Med. 2002; 347(14):1057-67.*

#19

Regarding the pharmacokinetics/pharmacodynamics of acetaminophen, which of the following statements are TRUE?

(Choose three answers.)

A. Following ingestion, approximately 4% of the ingested acetaminophen is excreted unchanged in the urine, while the remainder is metabolized in the liver.

B. Adults and children metabolize acetaminophen in an identical fashion, utilizing the sulfation and glucuronidation pathways to equivalent degrees.

C. After metabolism in the liver, the remainder of acetaminophen is metabolized via the P450 isoenzyme to form NAPQI.

D. The human body normally has enough glutathione to reduce NAPQI, which results in renal excretion of cysteine and mercapturic acid conjugates.

E. The half life of acetaminophen is approximately 12 hours.

#19

Answer: A, C, and D

In adults, 45-55% of acetaminophen is glucuronidated, while 20-30% is sulfated. In pediatric patients, however, sulfation is the primary pathway, and glucuronidation is a minor component. The remainder of acetaminophen is metabolized by P450 to NAPQI, and usually our body's endogenous glutathione supplies are able to bind and reduce NAPQI. In toxicity, the amount of NAPQI exceeds the endogenous supply and hepatotoxicity results. Acetaminophen has a half-life of 1.5-2.5 hours, although it can be slightly prolonged at supratherapeutic concentrations.

- *Rosen's Emergency Medicine - Concepts and Clinical Practice. 8th edition. 2013. Chapter 148: Acetaminophen. 1960-1964.*

#20

Regarding acetaminophen-induced hepatotoxicity, the greatest risk factor for hepatotoxicity is:

A. Acute ethanol intoxication

B. Chronic ethanol abuse

C. Prolonged time from ingestion to administration of N-acetylcysteine

D. Pediatric age

#20

Answer: C

Anything that induces the P450 isoenzyme can theoretically increased the risk for acetaminophen-induced hepatotoxicity. One of the best-studied agents for inducing P450 is ethanol. Thus, chronic ethanol consumption leads to increased P450 activity and subsequently increases the risk of hepatotoxicity during an acute ingestion. In contrast, the co-ingestion of ethanol with acetaminophen in a non-alcoholic may result in inhibition of the oxidation of acetaminophen, thereby providing some degree of protection from hepatotoxicity during acute acetaminophen ingestion. The strongest risk factor for developing hepatotoxicity, however, is the time from a toxic ingestion until NAC is started. The risk is low if NAC is started within the first 6-8 hours, while the risk increases substantially with delays longer than 8 hours. Pediatric patients appear to be somewhat resistant to acetaminophen induced hepatotoxicity when compared with adults. The increased rate of sulfation and the increased relative size of the liver may be protective.

- *Rosen's Emergency Medicine - Concepts and Clinical Practice. 2013. Chapter 148: Acetaminophen. 1960-1964.*

#21

Regarding acetaminophen toxicity, which of the following statements are TRUE?

(Choose two answers.)

    A. Any detectable acetaminophen 24 hours or more after ingestion is an indication for treatment (with the right clinical scenario).

    B. Syrup of ipecac should be administered when the patient arrives to the ED if the ingestion was within the last hour.

    C. Since charcoal absorbs NAC, charcoal gastrointestinal decontamination is contraindicated.

    D. NAC acts as a free radical scavenger and a glutathione substrate.

    E. The original oral NAC regimen has a shorter duration of treatment than IV NAC.

#21
Answer: A and D

The nomogram (Rumack-Matthew) uses a threshold of 150 mcg/ml at four hours after ingestion and 75 mcg/ml at 8 hours after ingestion as a threshold for treatment. Any detectable acetaminophen at 24 hours or more after ingestion is an indication for treatment, in the right clinical scenario. There is no role for Ipecac in the ED management of acetaminophen ingestion or any over-dose. Similarly, gastric lavage is not indicated in acet-aminophen ingestion, as the risks outweigh the benefits. Some have raised concern that NAC will be absorbed by the charcoal, thus yielding suboptimal concentrations of NAC. However, it has been demonstrated that the ab-sorption rate is of minimal clinical consequence. NAC acts as a free radical scavenger and a glutathione sub-strate. The oral NAC regimen takes 72 hours to complete. In 2004, the FDA approved the IV formulation, which in-volves 150 mg/kg over 1 hour, followed by 12.5 mg/kg/hr for 4 hours, followed by 6.25 mg/kg/hr for 16 hrs (= 21 hours).

- *Rosen's Emergency Medicine - Concepts and Clinical Practice. 8th edition. 2013. Chapter 148: Acetaminophen. 1960-1964.*

#22

It is now 5:00 PM. You are seeing a patient who states that he took 20 pills of acetaminophen at 12:00 PM (5 hours before) and then took another few pills at 3:00PM (2 hours before). When should the blood be drawn to be able to apply the Rumack-Matthew nomogram?

    A. Now – 5:00 PM

    B. At 7:00 PM

    C. Never

    D. 9:00 PM

    E. Serially, every hour for 4 hours

#22

Answer: A

It is important to recall that the Rumack-Matthew nomogram was designed to assess the acetaminophen level after a single, acute ingestion. Unfortunately, many times, patients do not present after a single acute ingestion, but rather consume some pills and a few hours later consume additional pills. In this case, to use the nomogram, the safest method is to assume that all pills were ingested at the first time, and plot the level based on that time. In coordination with the poison control center a later repeat acetaminophen level could be drawn.

- *Rosen's Emergency Medicine - Concepts and Clinical Practice. 8th edition. 2013. Chapter 148: Acetaminophen. 1960-1964.*

#23

A patient is transferred from psychiatry because they are concerned that he ingested acetaminophen. Unfortunately, the patient refuses to reveal when he took the pills, or if he even took any pills. You obtain an acetaminophen level, and it is not detectable, and LFTs and INR are normal. You should:

    A. Start NAC treatment.

    B. Recheck LFTs and INR and acetaminophen level in 2 hours.

    C. Do nothing.

#23

Answer: C

Not uncommonly, patients will present with an un-known time of ingestion. Occasionally, this is because the patient is non-compliant, but more often, this occurs in mixed ingestions in which the patient is encephalo-pathic or intubated and therefore unable to provide any history. In these cases, an acetaminophen level, liver tests, and an INR should be ordered. If there is no detect-able Tylenol, and liver and INR tests are normal, then no treatment is indicated for Tylenol ingestion. If there is any detectable Tylenol, or elevated transaminases or PT, then NAC treatment is indicated. Chronic ingestions in which the patients have taken supratherapeutic in-gestions for several days should be managed the same as when the time of ingestion is unknown.

It is also important to assess if the patient is still suicidal and will attempt another ingestion.

- *Rosen's Emergency Medicine - Concepts and Clinical Practice. 8th edition. 2013. Chapter 148: Acetaminophen. 1960-1964.*

#24

A 32 year old G3P2 patient who is 20 weeks by dates presents after a acetaminophen ingestion. TRUE statements about acetaminophen in pregnancy include which of the following?

A. Acetaminophen does not cross the placenta.

B. Acetaminophen is a teratogen.

C. N-acetylcysteine does not cross the placenta.

D. The Rumack-Matthew nomogram should be adjusted in pregnancy.

E. The management is the same for pregnant and non-pregnant patients.

#24

Answer: E

Acetaminophen readily crosses the placenta, which places the fetus at risk for hepatotoxicity. However, NAPQI does not cross the placenta, and thus, the fetus must metabolize the acetaminophen for toxicity to occur. The fetus is able to start metabolizing acetaminophen into toxic and non-toxic metabolites at approximately 18 weeks of gestational age. NAC does cross the placenta and its use is indicated in pregnant women whose serum concentration is above the treatment line of the Rumack-Matthew nomogram. Fetal outcome appears to be worse with delays in commencing NAC.

- *Rosen's Emergency Medicine - Concepts and Clinical Practice. 8th edition. 2013. Chapter 148: Acetaminophen. 1960-1964.*

#25

You are treating a patient suspected of a acetamino-phen overdose with N-acetylcysteine (NAC) intraven-ously. The patient develops mild flushing. What should be done?

A. Treat with diphenhydramine.

B. Treat with steroids.

C. Treat with bronchodilators.

D. All of the above

E. None of the above

#25

Answer: E

Allergic and anaphylactoid reactions are known side effects of IV NAC therapy. If flushing is the only symptom, the NAC infusion should be held for 1 hour and restarted at a slower rate. Patients with urticaria should be treated with diphenhydramine. Those with angioedema, hypotension, or respiratory symptoms (e.g., bronchospasm) should be treated with diphenhydramine, corticosteroids, and bronchodilators for bronchospasm. If a patient can tolerate oral NAC, then therapy can also be switched from the IV to oral route. In children given an incorrect dose, adverse effects can include cerebral edema and hyponatremia (due to administration in 5% dextrose). There are rare reports of deaths due to anaphylactoid reactions from NAC therapy.

. *Heard KJ. Acetylcysteine for acetaminophen poisoning. N Engl J Med. 2008 Jul 17; 359(3): 285-92. full text*

#26

Acetaminophen is absorbed rapidly, with peak plasma concentration generally occurring within ____ hours and complete absorption within _____ hours?

A. 1, 4

B. 2, 8

C. 3, 10

D. 4, 12

E. 6, 12

#26

Answer: A

Acetaminophen is absorbed rapidly with peak plasma concentrations generally within 1 hour and complete absorption within 4 hours. Once absorbed, acetaminophen inhibits PGE2 synthesis, leading to antipyresis and analgesia. The 4-hour mark is important because this is what treatment should be based on, according to the nomogram. If the serum concentration level is greater than 150 micrograms/liter at 4 hours, then antidotal treatment with N-acetylcysteine should be started.e:

- *Rosen's Emergency Medicine - Concepts and Clinical Practice. 8th edition. 2013. Chapter 148: Acetaminophen. 1960-1964.*

#27

General considerations for latrodectus antivenin (black widow spider bite antivenom) include which of the following:

   A. Patients with seizures as a result of the envenomation

   B. Respiratory failure

   C. Uncontrolled hypertension

   D. Pregnant women

   E. All of the above

#27

Answer: E

In general, pediatric patients, pregnant women and the elderly may need to be given latrodectus antivenin (Lyovac), which is derived from horse serum. Clinical judgment must be used to adjust for the age and category of patients needing antivenin. Antivenin should be administered to patients with severe envenomation manifested as seizures, respiratory failure, or uncontrolled hypertension with end-organ damage; to symptomatic pregnant women; and to patients not responding to other analgesic therapy. Treatment for black widow spider bites consists of applying ice packs to the bite area for relief of pain and observing for 6 hours for other worsening symptoms.

- *Rosen's Emergency Medicine - Concepts and Clinical Practice. 8th edition. 2013. Chapter 62: Venomous Animal Injuries. 803-804.*

#28

True statements about gamma-hydroxybutyrate (GHB) intoxication include all of the following EXCEPT:

A. GHB is detected on most urine toxicology screens.

B. Patients who suddenly stop GHB or its precursors after chronic, frequent use can experience a severe and potentially life-threatening withdrawal syndrome.

C. Rapid recovery from coma or periods of agitation alternating with periods of decreased level of consciousness is characteristic.

D. Eye examination may reveal miosis with or without nystagmus.

E. Hypothermia may occur.

#28
Answer: A

GHB is not detected on most urine toxicology screens. If laboratory confirmation is required, specimens must be collected early to capture the parent compound, and gas chromatography-mass spectroscopy must be performed. The drug may be detected in urine up to 12 hours after ingestion. Rapid recovery from coma, or periods of agitation alternating with periods of decreased level of consciousness is characteristic. Hypothermia may occur, and eye examination may reveal miosis with or without nystagmus. A distinctive feature of GHB intoxication is respiratory depression with apnea, interrupted by periods of agitation and combativeness. Emesis, seizures, and myoclonus may be present. Similar to other sedatives and hypnotics, patients who suddenly stop GHB can experience a severe withdrawal syndrome.

- *Rosen's Emergency Medicine - Concepts and Clinical Practice. 8th edition. 2013. Chapter 165: Sedative Hypnotics. 2082-2083.*

- *Goldfrank's Toxicologic Emergencies 10th edition. 2014. Chapter 83: Gamma-Hydroxybutyric Acid.*

#29

You are seeing a patient who admits to ingesting salicylates in a suicide gesture. Indications for dialysis include which of the following?

(Choose three answers.)

    A. Salicylate level of 50 mg/dL

    B. Seizure and coma

    C. Renal failure

    D. Pulmonary edema

#29

Answer: B, C, and D

Hemodialysis is recommended in patients with the following:

1. Serum salicylate levels greater than 100 mg/dL in acute intoxication and 50 mg/dL in chronic poisoning
2. Altered mental status
3. Respiratory failure
4. Coma
5. Renal or hepatic failure
6. Pulmonary edema
7. Severe acid-base disturbance
8. Failure to respond (refractory acidemia) to conservative treatment.

• *Rosen's Emergency Medicine - Concepts and Clinical Practice. 8th edition. 2013. Chapter 149: Aspirin and NSAIDS. 1965-1967.*

#30

You are treating a patient with salicylate toxicity and you are trying to alkalinize the urine to a pH of 7.5 to 8.0. Despite increasing the bicarbonate in the IVF the pH will not rise above 6.0. What electrolyte might be responsible?

A. Sodium

B. Potassium

C. Calcium

D. Chloride

#30

Answer: B

Alkaline urine traps the salicylate ion and increases excretion. Urinary alkalinization is recommended in patients with levels greater than 35 mg/dL. A urine pH of 7.5-8.0 is necessary to increase excretion. Urinary alkalinization is difficult to achieve because the excretion of salicylic acid in the urine decreases urinary pH. Additionally, hypokalemia must be corrected to attain an alkaline urine. Alkaline urine should NOT be produced at the cost of systemic acidemia. Forced diuresis does not significantly increase salicylate excretion and may potentiate cerebral and pulmonary edema.

- *Rosen's Emergency Medicine - Concepts and Clinical Practice. 8th edition. 2013. Chapter 149: Aspirin and NSAIDS. 1965-1967.*

#31

True or False: In a patient with NSAID overdose, urinary alkalinization should be initiated, and if this fails, hemodialysis should be initiated.

    A. True

    B. False

#31

Answer: B

NSAID overdose is usually self-limited, with predominantly gastrointestinal toxicity and treatment is usually just supportive. Pyrazolones and fenamates can cause seizures, though. There is no evidence for activated charcoal. Because of the high protein metabolism, urinary alkalinization, hemodialysis, or hemoperfusion is not usually useful. Multi-dose activated charcoal reduces the elimination half-life of phenylbutazone by 30% and may be beneficial in cases of severe intoxication.

- *Rosen's Emergency Medicine - Concepts and Clinical Practice. 8th edition. 2013. Chapter 149: Aspirin and NSAIDS. 1967-1969.*

TRAUMA AND SURGERY

#1

Regarding blunt traumatic aortic injury, which of the following statements is FALSE?

A. The majority of tears occur in the ascending aorta.

B. The possibility of aortic disruption must be considered in every patient who sustains a severe deceleration injury.

C. The most common symptom is interscapular or retrosternal pain.

D. An increase in the width of the superior mediastinum is the most sensitive sign and is found in 50% to 92% of aortic ruptures, but specificity of this sign is 10%.

E. Helical CT has almost 100% sensitivity and specificity for detecting aortic rupture.

#1

Answer: A

The majority of aortic tears (80-90%) occur in the descending aorta at the isthmus, just distal to the left subclavian artery. Other, less common sites of involvement are the ascending aorta, the distal descending aorta at the level of the diaphragm, the mid-thoracic descending aorta, and the origin of the left subclavian artery. Patients commonly present with scapular or back pain, although this has poor sensitivity.

Depending on the location of the injury, signs and symptoms can include, tracheal compression and deviation, stridor or hoarseness caused by compression of the laryngeal nerve, dysphagia from esophageal compression, and extremity pain caused by ischemia from decreased arterial flow.

An increase in the superior mediastinum is the most sensitive sign (50-92%), but it is poorly specific (10%). Other causes of mediastinal widening include venous bleeding from the clavicle, thoracic spine, or sternum, as well as from pulmonary contusions, and mediastinal masses.

- *Rosen's Emergency Medicine - Concepts and Clinical Practice. 8th edition. 2013. Chapter 45: Thoracic Trauma. 451-454.*

#2

Which of the following statements is FALSE regarding the management of the adult patient with blunt abdominal trauma?

A. CT of the abdomen and pelvis with oral and IV contrast can exclude bowel, diaphragm, and pancreatic injuries.

B. CT with oral contrast is not essential to the evaluation of blunt abdominal trauma.

C. Diagnostic peritoneal lavage (DPL) can be used to exclude hemoperitoneum.

D. DPL does not define the extent of injury.

E. DPL has a 1-2% complication rate and may lead to non-therapeutic laparotomies.

Amy Kaji

#2

Answer: A

CT can not exclude bowel, diaphragm, and pancreatic injuries. Sensitivity of CT scan for pancreatic injuries has been reported to be as low as 30%, and for diaphragmatic injuries, as low as 61%. Due to the limitations of DPL, current consensus recommendations include FAST and CT for the initial evaluation of blunt abdominal trauma.

- *Clinical Policy: Critical Issues in the Evaluation of Adult Patients Presenting to the Emergency Department with Acute Blunt Abdominal Trauma. Ann Emerg Med. 2011 Apr; 57(4): 387-404. full text*

#3

Which of the following are indications to obtain CT angiography to screen for blunt carotid and vertebral injuries?

(Choose three answers.)

    A. C1-C3 fracture

    B. C-spine fracture with subluxation

    C. Fractures involving the foramen transversarium

    D. Isolated seatbelt sign

    E. Hematoma to the posterior neck

#3

Answer: A, B, and C

Studies have shown that specific fracture patterns have high associations with carotid and vertebral injuries:

1. Patients presenting with any neurologic abnormality that is unexplained by a diagnosed injury

2. Blunt trauma patients presenting with epistaxis from a suspected arterial source after trauma

3. Glasgow Coma Scale score ≤ 8

4. Petrous bone fracture

5. Diffuse axonal injury

6. Cervical spine fracture particularly those with fracture of C1 to C3 and fracture through the foramen transversarium

7. Cervical spine fracture with subluxation or rotational component

8. Lefort II or III facial fractures

Pediatric trauma patients should be evaluated using the same criteria as the adult population.

The Eastern Association for Surgery and Trauma recommend routine screening for vascular injury in these patients with these fracture patterns.

•   Bromberg WJ et al. Blunt cerebrovascular injury practice management guidelines: the Eastern Association for the Surgery of Trauma. J Trauma. 2010 Feb; 68(2): 471-7. full text

#4

Which of the following has been found to be harmful in the management of the adult patient with severe head trauma?

A. Avoiding hypoxia

B. Corticosteroids

C. Avoiding extreme hyperventilation and hypocarbia

D. Avoiding hypotension

E. Anti-seizure prophylaxis

#4

Answer: B

MRC CRASH was a randomized controlled trial of the effect of corticosteroids on death and disability after head injury. The investigators randomly allocated 10,008 adults with head injury and a Glasgow Coma Scale score of 14 or less, within 8 h of injury, to a 48-h infusion of corticosteroid (methylprednisolone) or placebo. Data at 6 months were obtained for 9673 (96.7%) patients. The risk of death was higher in the corticosteroid group than in the placebo group (1248 [25.7%] vs 1075 [22.3%] deaths; relative risk 1.15, 95% CI 1.07-1.24; p=0.0001), as was the risk of death or severe disability. There was no evidence that the effect of corticosteroids differed by injury severity or time since injury. Thus, the authors concluded that corticosteroids should not be used routinely in the treatment of head injury.

•   Roberts I, et al. The effect of corticosteroids on death within 14 days 10008 adult patients with clinically significant head injury; MRC CRASH trial: randomized controlled trial. Lancet. 2004; 364 (9442): 1321-1328.

#5

Regarding penetrating neck trauma, which of the following statement is FALSE?

A. Zone II injuries are the most common and cause the highest mortality rate.

B. Zone I defines the region from the clavicles to the inferior rim of the cricoid cartilage.

C. Zone II spans the region from the superior edge of the cricoid to the angle of the mandible.

D. Zone III extends superiorly from the angle of the mandible to the base of the skull.

E. The platysma is an important landmark in gauging the severity of a wound, with violation indicating potential injury to underlying structures.

#5

Answer: A

Zone I defines the region between the clavicles and the inferior rim of the cricoid cartilage. The structures potentially injured in Zone 1 of the neck include:

1. Common carotid artery
2. Subclavian artery
3. Vertebral body
4. Apex of lung
5. Distal trachea and esophagus
6. Thoracic Duct
7. Thyroid

Although zone II injuries are the most common, zone I injuries are associated with the greatest mortality due to difficulty in achieving control of the vasculature and need to enter the thoracic cavity.

• *Rosen's Emergency Medicine - Concepts and Clinical Practice. 8th edition. 2013. Chapter 44: Neck. 422-428.*

#6

You are faced with a victim of self-inflicted hanging/ strangulation. Which of the following are appropriate management steps?

A. Monitor the airway and perform intubation early if needed.

B. Obtain early ENT consultation for suspected laryngotracheal injuries.

C. Consider the possibility of increased ICP in patients with a depressed sensorium.

D. Obtain early neurosurgical consultation if there is any evidence of increased intracranial pressure.

E. Address psychiatric or social issues that after stabilization and control of injuries.

F. All of the above

#6

Answer: F

All of the statements are true. The clinical presentation of a patient with a strangulation injury can vary from hemodynamic stability to a full cardiac arrest, and from normal mental status to coma. The presenting mental status and GCS are related to the duration of the hanging, but the GCS is a poor predictor of the patient's final outcome. Patients presenting with a low GCS have survived the injury with normal mental status. The major causes of mortality from strangulation are asphyxia, spinal cord injuries, arterial occlusion, and cardiac arrest.

- *Rosen's Emergency Medicine - Concepts and Clinical Practice. 8th edition. 2013. Chapter 44: Neck. 422-428.*

#7

Regarding the neurologic examination after a trauma, the following are true, EXCEPT:

A. Hemiparesis contralateral to a fixed and dilated pupil suggests herniation.

B. Decorticate posturing is abnormal flexion of the upper extremity and extension of the lower extremity.

C. Decerebrate posturing is associated with a better prognosis than decorticate posturing.

D. Decerebrate posturing results in abnormal extension and adduction of the arms with internal rotation.

E. False localizing signs for the motor examination can also be caused by occult extremity trauma, spinal cord injury, or nerve root injury that makes the examination painful or difficult.

#7

Answer: C

Decerebrate posturing indicates brain stem damage, specifically damage below the level of the red nucleus and generally portends a poor prognosis. Decerebrate posturing is also called extensor posturing. All of the other statements are true.

- *Rosen's Emergency Medicine - Concepts and Clinical Practice. 8th edition. 2013. Chapter 41: Head Injuries. 346.*

#8
Which of the following statements is FALSE?

A. Brainstem activity can be assessed by a patient's respiratory pattern, pupillary size, and eye movements.

B. The oculocephalic response (doll's eyes maneuver) tests the integrity of the pontine gaze centers.

C. The oculovestibular response (cold water calorics) assesses the brainstem.

D. Comatose patients will demonstrate nystagmus when cold water is instilled in the ear canal.

E. In the severely head-injured patient, the cranial nerve examination is often limited to the pupillary response, gag reflex, and corneal reflex.

Amy Kaji

#8

Answer: D

When cold water is instilled into the ear canal, a comatose patient will not have nystagmus. Instead, eyes will tonically deviate toward the side of cold water. All of the other statements are all true.

- *Rosen's Emergency Medicine - Concepts and Clinical Practice. 8th edition. 2013. Chapter 41: Head Injuries. 347-346.*

#9

Head trauma can produce profound effects on the cardiovascular system from:

    A. The amount of blood loss within the cranial cavity

    B. The destruction of the hypothalamic-pituitary axis

    C. Compression of the brainstem and medulla, which can cause cardiac instability

    D. A basilar skull fracture and CSF leakage

    E. Ischemia to the astrocytes

#9

Answer: C

Head trauma can produce profound effects on the cardio-vascular system if compression of the brainstem and medulla occur and produce cardiac instability. The amount of blood lost within the cranium should not cause hemodynamic instability from a volume standpoint. All head injured patients should have cardiac monitoring when they are transported.

- *Rosen's Emergency Medicine - Concepts and Clinical Practice. 8th edition. 2013. Chapter 41: Head Injuries. 348-49, 361.*

#10
Which of the following would be considered patterns of NON occlusive vascular injury from trauma?

(Choose two answers.)

    A. Transection

    B. Thrombosis

    C. Reversible spasm

    D. Arteriovenous fistula

    E. Pseudoaneurysm

#10

Answer: D and E

Examples of non occlusive injury include intimal flaps, arteriovenous fistulas, and pseudo-aneurysms. Occlusive injury trauma patterns include transection, thrombosis, and reversible spasm.

- *Rosen's Emergency Medicine - Concepts and Clinical Practice. 8th edition. 2013. Chapter 48: Peripheral Vascular Injuries. 507.*

#11

A motorcyclist presents after a high speed accident. His exam is significant for severe left calf pain and swelling. X-rays show a midshaft tibial fracture. Given his exquisite pain, swelling, and loss of distal sensation, you are concerned for a compartment syndrome. What minimal compartment pressure would indicate the need for fasciotomy?

    A. 10 mm Hg

    B. 15 mm Hg

    C. 20 mm Hg

    D. 30 mm Hg

    E. 45 mm Hg

#11

Answer: D

Compartment Syndrome is often associated with a closed long bone fracture of the tibia but is well described in the thigh, forearm, arm, hand and foot. As tissue pressure increases, venous pressure increases which compromises the local circulation and causes tissue hypoxia. It is thought to occur at pressures that are above normal diastolic pressure but below systemic arterial pressure because of a reduced arteriovenous gradient. Normal compartment pressure is 0 mm Hg. Circulation begins to be impaired when tissue pressures reach 30 mm Hg or more.

Although no finding is universally present in compartment syndrome, some findings that should suggest the diagnosis are:

1. Pain out of proportion to injury
2. Pain on passive extension of flexion
3. Paresthesia
4. Changes in skin color
5. Loss of distal pulses

Pressures greater than 30mm Hg or within 30 mm Hg of the diastolic pressure are indications of fasciotomy in the correct clinical setting.

- *Rosen's Emergency Medicine - Concepts and Clinical Practice. 8th edition. 2013. Chapter 49: General Principles of Orthopedic Injuries. 519-525.*

#12

You are caring for a patient who was involved in a high speed MVA with blunt head trauma from the steering wheel. Upon return from the CT scanner, you note his right eye is swollen with chemosis. As you stand at the head of the bed, his right eye appears slightly proptotic. Visual acuity is OS 20/20 and OD 20/100. The radiologist notifies you of a retrobulbar hemorrhage on the right. Which of the following is FALSE regarding this patient's condition?

A. You should confirm that there is no evidence of globe rupture since that would be a contraindication to lateral canthotomy.

B. Visual acuity and IOP should be measured (after globe rupture is excluded).

C. Lateral canthotomy should be performed within one hour of injury to avoid permanent vision loss.

D. Chemosis, proptosis, asymmetry of globe, ophthalmoplegia, and elevated IOP are findings consistent with acute orbital compartment syndrome.

E. Visual acuity should return to normal immediately after canthotomy and should therefore be remeasured to assess for efficacy of the procedure.

Amy Kaji

#12

Answer E

The orbit is composed of 7 bones that enclose all but the anterior aspect. The globe obstructs the opening to the bony orbit. Following trauma, the presence of hemorrhage, foreign body, or edema can increase retrobulbar pressure leading to an elevation of intraocular pressure. Immediately following a lateral canthotomy, the intraocular pressure elevation should resolve. However, any pupillary defect and visual acuity may not resolve immediately, but rather, over hours. The only contraindication to performing a lateral canthotomy is an open globe.

• *Rosen's Emergency Medicine - Concepts and Clinical Practice. 8th edition. 2013. Chapter 42: Facial Trauma. 379-80.*

. *McInnes G, Howes DW. Lateral canthotomy and cantholysis: a simple, vision-saving procedure. CJEM. 2002; 4(1): 49-52. full text*

#13

A 30 year old male presents to the ED after sustaining an injury while mountain biking. After landing his bicycle following a jump over a log, his feet slipped out of the pedals and he straddled the crossbar. He complains of dysuria and hematuria. Your examination finds a stable pelvis, no penile or testicular trauma but a tender perineal hematoma. The urine specimen is grossly bloody and there is blood at the meatus. Which of the following is FALSE regarding management of this patient?

A. Given the mechanism and physical findings, your suspicion for a lower GU (bladder/urethral injury) injury is high.

B. Given ongoing hematuria, a foley catheter should be placed in order to tamponade any injury and to control blood loss.

C. Retrograde urethrogram is the diagnostic procedure of choice in detecting urethral injury and can be used to evaluate bladder trauma.

D. Urethral injury is suggested by the presence of a pelvic fracture or evidence of a scrotal hematoma.

E. If a partial urethral injury is discovered on retrograde urethrogram, one careful attempt to pass a 12- or 14-Fr foley or coude catheter may be undertaken.

#13

Answer: B

Urethral injury is suggested by the presence of a pelvic fracture, blood at the urethral meatus, presence of a high-riding, absent prostate on rectal exam, or evidence of a perineal/scrotal/penile hematoma. Abdominal tenderness, pelvic instability or tenderness to palpation should raise your concern for pelvic fracture and potential lower urinary tract injury. Gross blood at the meatus is diagnostic of urethral injury and dictates evaluation by retrograde urethrography.

A foley catheter should never be introduced when there is suspected urethral trauma without first ensuring integrity by retrograde urethrography. Failure to do this may convert a partial urethral tear into a complete disruption. Retrograde urethrography should be performed in evaluation of any lower GU injury. If a partial urethral injury is discovered , one careful attempt to pass a 12- or 14 Fr foley or coude catheter may be undertaken.

· *Rosen's Emergency Medicine - Concepts and Clinical Practice. 8th edition. 2013. Chapter 47: Genitourinary System. 481-489.*

#14

You are caring for an auto vs. pedestrian trauma patient. In the field, the patient's blood pressure is 92/70 with a HR of 101. On arrival to the ED, his blood pressure is 85/60 and HR 115. Your primary survey reveals an unstable pelvis and lower abdominal tenderness. No further injuries are discovered. What would be the LEAST appropriate initial management for this patient?

A. Crystalloid infusion and blood transfusion

B. External fixator device (T-Pod or bedsheet)

C. Angiography and vessel embolization if there is no fluid on FAST and patient's pelvis is stabilized

D. FAST exam or DPL

E. Immediate thoracotomy and aortic cross-clamping

#14

Answer: E

In evaluation of patients with pelvic fracture and blunt abdominal trauma, hemodynamic stability should be primarily assessed. If the patient is stable, intraperitoneal injury can be evaluated by CT. However, in cases in which the patient is hemodynamically unstable, the presence of intraperitoneal hemorrhage directs therapy and management. In an unstable patient, a positive ultrasound/FAST exam finding is consistent with intraperitoneal hemorrhage and the need for emergent laparotomy. In the absence of intraperitoneal hemorrhage in blunt abdominal trauma with pelvic fracture and hemodynamic instability, pelvic fracture stabilization and angiography/embolization is warranted. Retroperitoneal bleeding can be massive and life threatening after pelvic fracture. Up to 4 L of blood can be held in the retroperitoneal space. Laparotomy is used only as a last resort because opening the abdominal cavity can relieve a tamponade and cause further hemorrhage.

- *Rosen's Emergency Medicine - Concepts and Clinical Practice. 8th edition. 2013. Chapter 46: Abdominal Trauma. 361-370.*

#15

The following patients are brought in to the ED with C-collars in place. Which patients, if any, could have their cervical spines cleared clinically and removed from immobilization?

(Choose two answers.)

A. 9 year old female with unwitnessed fall from bed onto carpeted floor with no loss of consciousness or neck pain, ambulating on scene upon paramedic arrival and only complains of an abrasion to the elbow and tingling/pins and needles sensation in her hand.

B. 47 year old male who was assaulted with loss of consciousness, with GCS 4-6-5, with no other injury/deficits.

C. 18 year old male who is alert and oriented with facial abrasions but with no neurological deficits, loss of consciousness or neck pain brought in after an MVA in which his main injury is an open femur fracture.

D. 27 year old intoxicated female found down outside of a bar GCS 4-6-4 initially upon paramedic arrival now 4-6-5.

E. 95 year old woman who sustained a mechanical fall in bathtub. No midline neck pain, alert and oriented, with no other complaints/injuries, and a normal neurologic exam.

#15

Answer B and E

A prospective observational study involving 34,069 trauma patients at 21 trauma centers in the U.S. validated a clinical decision instrument (NEXUS) for identifying patients of extremely low probability for spinal injury. Sensitivity 99.6%, Negative predictive value 99.8%. Specificity 12.9%, Positive predictive value 2.7%. Patients must fulfill all five criteria to be classified as low probability for C-spine injury and thus have a clinically cleared C-spine:

1. No midline cervical tenderness
2. No focal neurological deficit
3. Normal alertness
4. No intoxication
5. No painful or distracting injury.

• *Hoffman JR, et al. Validity of a set of clinical criteria to rule out injury to the cervical spine in patients with blunt trauma. National Emergency X-Radiography Utilization Study Group. N Engl J Med. 2000; 343(2): 94-9. full text*

#16

A six year old female playing on a jungle gym is reported to have fallen from the slide striking her head on the ground. Which of the following would be most concerning in terms of symptoms/signs of increased intracranial pressure?

A. If the patient had a tonic-clonic seizure immediately after impacting the ground lasting 1 minute; GCS 15 upon paramedic arrival.

B. If the patient has an single episode of vomiting approximately 10 minutes after injury while being loaded into the ambulance.

C. If the patient complains of a persistent headache.

D. If the patient was crying after the event.

#16

Answer: C

In pediatric trauma, it is helpful to clearly determine whether there was loss of consciousness at the time of injury. Transient pallor, irritability, diaphoresis, emesis (not persistent) may be reported with minor trauma. A brief seizure that occurs immediately after the insult with rapid return to normal level of conscious is considered an impact seizure and doesn't mandate neurosurgical evaluation or anticonvulsant therapy. Seizures occurring more than 20 minutes after the event portend a greater possibility of traumatic brain injury and warrant further evaluation/CT imaging. Common symptoms and signs of increased ICP in pediatrics include persistent headache, neck stiffness, photophobia, altered mental status, persistent emesis, cranial nerve involvement, papilledema, hypertension, bradycardia, hypoventilation, and posturing.

- *Rosen's Emergency Medicine - Concepts and Clinical Practice. 8th edition. 2013. Chapter 41: Head Injuries 341-344.*

#17

A three-year old boy is brought in by paramedics for burns to his face, neck, chest, arms, and hands after pulling down a pot of hot water from the stove. His primary exam is negative, and his secondary exam is significant for 15% BSA second degree partial thickness burns and 10% first degree burns. You initiate a trauma activation, look for concomitant injuries, and administer the proper dose of analgesics. You want to calculate his fluid requirements as you prepare to transfer him to a burn center. He is 15 kilograms, White on the Broselow. His vital signs are now normal. You calculate the Parkland formula for the next few hours, and add this quantity to the required maintenance fluids and elect to give:

A. 450mL over the next eight hours = 56 mL/hour

B. 450 over the next eight hours = 56 mL/hour + 50mL/hour (maintenance fluids) = 106 mL/hour

C. NS bolus of 20 mL/kg = 300 mL over next 30-45 minutes only

D. D5 ½ NS with 20 mEq KCL at 50 mL/hour

E. Start a PO challenge and observe oral tolerance before calculating IV fluids.

#17

Answer: B

The Parkland formula aids in the calculation of initial fluid requirements in severely burned patients. Only second and third degree burns are considered in its calculation. The formula is 4 mL/kg x % BSA. Half of this amount is given over the first eight hours, the second half over the next 16 hours. In this case, 4 mL x 15 kg x 15% BSA = 900 mL. Half of this - 450 mL - is to be given over the next eight hours: 450 mL/8 hours = 56 mL/hour.

The Parkland formula underestimates the fluid requirements of young children, since it is based on weight, which corresponds imprecisely with BSA in growing children. In children younger than 5, the Parkland calculation should be added to the child's baseline maintenance needs. In this example, the Parkland formula yields 56 mL/hour; this, in addition to maintenance (15 kg child = 50 mL/hour) is a total of 106 mL/hour

(A) 56 mL/hour is the correct calculation for the Parkland formula only. This young child needs maintenance fluids in addition to the formula.

(C) NS bolus may be appropriate in the setting of trauma, but in this child with normal vital signs, it may not be necessary; in addition, the physician could easily "get behind" in this patient's fluid therapy by not anticipating his needs upfront.

(D) Although dextrose may be needed for young children in the setting of burns with documented hypoglycemia, burn patients should not receive potassium-containing fluids initially. The cellular breakdown associated with burns alone can cause the serum potassium to rise.

This boy meets multiple criteria for admission: partial thickness burn > 10% BSA, burn to face and hands.

- *Rosen's Emergency Medicine - Concepts and Clinical Practice. 8th edition. 2013. Chapter 63: Thermal Burns. 811-814.*

#18

Which patient(s) requires burn center/facility transfer?

A. 35 year old male with partial thickness burns to entire back, shoulders and buttocks

B. 23 year old female with circumferential full thickness burns to right hand and wrist

C. 55 year old male with circumferential partial thickness burns to entire right leg

D. 18 year old female after inhalation injury with multiple partial thickness burns and wheezing, with significant asthma history

E. A, B, C, and D

F. A and B

#18

Answer: E

Transfer guidelines for patients with severe burns include

- Any burn >10% of total body surface area (BSA) in patients <10 or >50 years old
- Burns involving >20% of total BSA in any patient
- Full thickness burns of hands, face, feet, genitalia, perineum or major joints
- Significant electrical injury
- Significant chemical injury
- Significant inhalation injury, concomitant mechanical trauma, pre-existing medical disorders
- Patients with special psychosocial or rehabilitative care needs

When a burn patient is being transferred to a burn center, early physician to physician contact with the burn center is essential. Prophylactic antibiotics are not indicated, and the use of antimicrobial creams on the burn wound should be postponed until admission to the burn center. Tetanus prophylaxis should be administered.

- *Rosen's Emergency Medicine - Concepts and Clinical Practice. 8th edition. 2013. Chapter 63: Thermal Burns. 811-814.*

- *Guidelines for the Operation of Burn Centers. Resources for Optimal Care of the Injured Patient 2006, Committee on Trauma, American College of Surgeons. 80-86. full text*

#19

A three-year old girl was poorly restrained during a high-speed motor vehicle collision. Her vital signs in the field were normal for age, her primary assessment is normal, and her secondary assessment is significant for swelling and ecchymosis around her left eye, and a lower lip laceration through the vermillion border. Regarding her potential injuries, which of the following is TRUE?

A. The decision to perform lateral canthotomy is based exclusively on mechanism of injury, regardless of lack of proptosis, chemosis, or vision loss.

B. The distance between the medial canthi of each eye should be no greater than the size of the palpebral fissure.

C. Iridodonesis refers to the bowing of the iris toward the pupil, indicating an iris root separation.

D. Cartilage tears of the ear heal well with minimal repair due to the robust blood supply to the head and neck.

#19

Answer: B

The distance between the medial canthi of each eye should be no greater than the size of the palpebral fissure. In other words, if the distance between the medial eye margins is larger than the length of the patient's eye, a midfacial fracture is likely. A careful physical examination will help to uncover other potential facial injuries, such as observation from the head of the bed (bird's eye view) and the foot of the bed (worm's eye view).

Lateral canthotomy is performed on clinical grounds. After severe blunt trauma, proptosis, vision loss, an afferent pupillary defect, chemosis, and increased intraocular pressure are all harbingers for rapid compression of the optic nerve due to retrobulbar hematoma.

Iridodonesis refers to the trembling movement of the iris after rapid eye movement, seen with lens dislocation. Iridodialysis is the separation of the iris root from the ciliary body; there is often a hyphema present, with complaints of glare, photophobia, or monocular diplopia.

Great care should be given to ear cartilage trauma. Cartilage is avascular, and defects must be repaired meticulously with overlying perichondrium, as well as with careful overlying soft tissue closure. Prophylactic antibiotics are recommended (especially for contaminated or devitalized wounds), and a compression dressing to prevent hematoma formation should be applied.

- *Rosen's Emergency Medicine - Concepts and Clinical Practice. 8th edition. 2013. Chapter 42: Facial Trauma. 379-380.*

#20

A six-year old girl is a restrained passenger wearing only a lap belt in a head-on collision, resulting in hyperflexion of her torso. She complains of abdominal pain and is uncomfortable on the backboard. Her injuries can be explained best by:

A. Waddell's Triad

B. Chance Fracture

C. Anxiety

D. Splenic laceration

#20

Answer: B

A Chance fracture can result from an improperly used lap belt. It is a hyperflexion fracture of a vertebral body, accompanied by hematoma or perforation of a loop of bowel. Often there is tenderness to palpation or an abdominal wall contusion is present.

Waddell's Triad is a constellation of injuries seen in pediatric pedestrian injury. The injury's include:

1. Femur fracture
2. Liver or splenic injury
3. Head trauma.

It is easy to remember by thinking through the events of an accident: The bumper of a car strikes the child in the thigh, causing femur (or pelvic) fracture, while the hood strikes the child in the flank, causing liver or splenic injury. The child is thrown through the air and lands head-first, sustaining brain injury. Although all three components are rarely present together, the concept of one injury associated with the others is important.

- *Rosen's Emergency Medicine - Concepts and Clinical Practice. 8th edition. 2013. Chapter 49: General Principles of Orthopedic Injuries. 512.*

Amy Kaji

#21

Regarding trauma in infants, which of the following is TRUE

A. A subgaleal hematoma is a collection of blood above the periosteum of the skull, while cephalo-hematomas form underneath the periosteum.

B. Cervical spine injury in infants is common, occurring in up to 10% of traumatized infants.

C. The American Academy of Pediatrics (AAP) has concise guidelines for imaging studies for infants with trauma, based on gestational age and results of skull plain films.

D. Due to the relatively compliant thoracic cage and underdeveloped musculature, the kidneys are the most commonly injured abdominal organ in infants.

#21

Answer: A

Infantile extracranial hematomas include:

1. Subgaleal hematoma – collection of blood between the galea aponeurotica and the periosteum. They are large, associated with skull fracture, and cross the suture lines.

2. Cephalohematoma – formation of blood underneath the periosteum; does not cross suture lines.

Cervical spine injuries in children are rare. Viccellio, et al. found that of 3065 pediatric patients who underwent imaging for a suspected head injury, less than 1% had cervical injury; none were under 2 years old.

The AAP has guidelines for blunt head trauma for children ages 2-20, based on an expert panel. The best evidence for determining the need for brain imaging in children is derived from the PECARN Pediatric Head Trauma Prediction Rules

The liver and spleen are the most frequently injured abdominal organs in infants, not the kidneys.

- *Rosen's Emergency Medicine - Concepts and Clinical Practice. 8th edition. 2013. Chapter 38: Pediatric Trauma. 312-13.*

- *Viccellio P, et al. A prospective multicenter study of cervical spine injury in children. Pediatrics. 2001 Aug; 108(2): e20.*

- *Kuppermann N, et al. Identification of children at very low risk of clinically-important brain injuries after head trauma: a prospective cohort study. The Lancet. 2009; 374(9696): 1160-1170. full text*

#22

64-year-old woman had a ground level fall and struck her her forehead. She had a brief convulsion immediately after the fall, and was unresponsive for less than 1 minute. When she awoke, she could not recall the event or the prior hour. She is now awake and oriented and had no abnormalities on neurologic examination. There is scalp tenderness and a contusion from the impact. Which of the following would NOT be indicated?

A. Head CT scan

B. Analgesics

C. Antiepileptic treatment

D. Counseling about post-concussion syndrome

E. Neuropsychological testing if impaired concentration persists after several weeks

#22

Answer: C

The patient in the vignette had a concussion complicated by an impact-related seizure, but had a normal neurologic examination. Since she is over the age of 60 and has obvious head trauma as well as amnesia, a CT scan should be obtained, according to the New Orleans and Canadian rules. After a normal examination and scan, she can be discharged with family. The patient should return if there is vomiting, confusion, weakness, or increased headache. There are no indications for antiseizure medication.

The patient should also be instructed about the sequela of concussion, so her expectations for recovery are appropriate. The patient may have headache, dizziness, and mild difficulty concentrating, which may persist for days or weeks. She should also be granted leave from work until concussive symptoms resolve. If impaired concentration persists for several weeks, neuropsychological testing should be considered.

- Ropper AH, et al. Concussion. N Engl J Med. 2007; 356:166-172. full text

#23

When comparing elder patients to younger patients in the NEXUS cohort, older patients had all the following EXCEPT:

A. They had a higher incidence of subdural hematomas.

B. They had a higher incidence of post-traumatic stress disorder.

C. They had a higher rate of contusions.

D. They had a higher rate of occult injuries.

E. They had a lower rate of basilar skull fractures.

#23
Answer: B

Rathlev NK, et al. reviewed all patients aged 65 years or older enrolled in the National Emergency X-Radiography Utilization Study (NEXUS) II head injury cohort. The authors assessed the prevalence and patterns of intracranial injuries among this cohort, and compared the prevalence of specific presenting signs and symptoms among injured and uninjured patients.

There were a total of 1,934 patients in this subgroup analysis (14.5% of NEXUS II patients).

Significant intracranial injury was defined as an injury that typically requires procedural intervention or is associated with persistent neurologic impairment or long-term disability. This occurred in 9.2% of elderly patients compared with 6.1% of non elderly patients. Focal neurologic deficits were present in 55.8% of those with injury. Those injuries included:

- Subdural hematoma
- Contusion
- Epidural hematoma
- Depressed skull fracture

Furthermore, 2.2% of elderly patients had an occult injury, compared with only 0.8% of younger patients.

The authors concluded that patients 65 years or older with head trauma are at higher risk of developing a significant intracranial injury, including subdural and epidural hematoma, with occult presentation being more common.

- *Rathlev NK, et al. Intracranial pathology in elders with blunt head trauma. Acad Emerg Med. 2006 Mar;13(3): 302-7. full text*

#24

You are seeing a patient with a traumatic brain injury, and the CT scan demonstrates an epidural hemorrhage (EDH). TRUE statements about EDH include which of the following:

(Choose three answers.)

A. EDH is a collection of blood between the dura mater and the skull.

B. EDH is less common in the very young (< 2 years old) than the elderly.

C. Epidural blood can be from venous or fracture bleeding.

D. EDH is classically lenticular in shape, smooth, and may cross the midline.

E. 100% of EDH are associated with a lucid interval.

#24

Answer: A, C, and D

EDH are less common in the very young (< 2 years old) than the elderly because of the close attachment of the dura to the skull. EDH classically occurs from a direct blow and rupture of the middle meningeal artery, but epidural blood also can be from venous or fracture bleeding. The lucid interval occurs in less than 50% of the time. The underlying brain parenchyma tends to be minimally interrupted, and the lesions are amenable to rapid surgical repair. EDH greater than 30 cm^3 in volume are generally evacuated regardless of the GCS.

- *Rosen's Emergency Medicine - Concepts and Clinical Practice. 8th edition. 2013. Chapter 41: Head Injury. 363.*

#25

Regarding traumatic brain injury (TBI), which of the following are recommended by the Brain Trauma Foundation?

(Choose two answers.)

    A. Prophylactic hyperventilation is recommended.

    B. Anticonvulsants can be used to decrease the incidence of early post-traumatic seizures.

    C. Fever is an independent predictor of poor outcome from TBI, so fevers should be treated.

    D. Head of bed should be lowered.

    E. Steroids are recommended for improving outcome and reducing ICP.

#25

Answer: B and C

Prophylactic hyperventilation is not recommended. Hyperventilation during the first 24 hours should be avoided while cerebral blood flow often is critically reduced. Hyperventilation is only recommended as a temporizing measure for the reduction of ICP.

The use of steroids is not recommended. In patients with TBI, high dose methylprednisolone is associated with increased mortality.

Anticonvulsants can be used early (1-7 days), as the reported incidence of early post-traumatic seizures ranges from 4-25%. Seizures can precipitate secondary brain injury by increasing ICP and decreasing oxygenation. However, early post-traumatic seizures are not associated with worse outcomes. Routine prophylaxis later than 1 week following TBI is not recommended.

Fever should be treated because it is an independent predictor of poor outcome from TBI.

Head of bed elevation to 30 degrees is recommended to lower ICP by facilitating venous drainage as well as CSF drainage through the foramen magnum. Reverse Trendelenburg can be used prior to spine clearance.

- *Rosen's Emergency Medicine - Concepts and Clinical Practice. 8th edition. 2013. Chapter 41: Head Injury. 349-351.*

- *Brain Trauma Foundation . Guidelines for the Management of Severe Traumatic Brain Injury. 3rd Edition. 2007. full text*

#26

You are seeing a 54 year old male, who fell 10 feet from a ladder and struck the back of his head. He is on warfarin for atrial fibrillation, and on examination his GCS is 1-4-2. TRUE statements about traumatic brain injury (TBI) include which of the following:

(Choose four answers.)

A. The two most important secondary insults to detect and reverse in TBI are hypercarbia and infection.

B. The two most important secondary insults to detect and reverse in TBI are hypoxia and hypotension.

C. Prehospital intubation of patients with severe TBI has not been found to consistently improve outcome.

D. Hypertension, alkalemia, and hypocapnia result in cerebral vasoconstriction and decreased cerebral blood flow (CBF).

E. Hypotension, acidemia, and hypercapnia result in vasodilation and increased cerebral blood flow.

#26

Answer: B - E

A single hypotensive measurement (according to data from the Traumatic Coma Data Bank) was independently associated with a doubling of mortality. Hypoxia (O2 sat < 90%) and fever (>100.4°F) are also associated with poor outcomes. While induced hypocapnia is used as a last ditch salvage technique during herniation, the potential benefit of routine prophylactic hypocapnia to prevent elevated ICP is greatly reduced by the harms of decreasing cerebral blood flow and subsequent ischemia.

Clinical efforts should be focused at minimizing secondary insults to the brain, including hypoxia, hypotension, hypocapnia, pyrexia, coagulopathy, and anemia. Several studies have suggested that prehospital RSI is associated with worse outcomes. The poor outcomes may be due to hypoxia during induction and inadvertent hyperventilation after intubation.

- *Rosen's Emergency Medicine - Concepts and Clinical Practice. 8th edition. 2013. Chapter 41: Head Injury. 340-342.*

- *Brain Trauma Foundation. Guidelines for the Management of Severe Traumatic Brain Injury. 3rd Edition. 2007. full text*

#27

Regarding traumatic brain injury (TBI) management, which of the following are TRUE with respect to what has been recommended by the Brain Trauma Foundation (BTF)?

    A. Blood pressure should be monitored and hypotension avoided.

    B. Aggressive attempts to maintain cerebral perfusion pressure (CPP) >70 mm Hg with fluids and vasopressors should be avoided because of the risk of ARDS.

    C. ICP should be monitored in all salvageable patients with severe TBI and an abnormal CT scan.

    D. ICP monitoring is indicated in patients with severe TBI, a normal CT scan, and two or more of the following: age >40 yo, motor posturing, or SBP <90 mm Hg.

    E. All of the above

#27

Answer: E

All are true. Both prehospital and in-hospital hypotension (SBP <90) have been implicated in poor outcomes. Hypotension is associated with a doubling of the mortality. A CPP < 50 should be avoided, and adequate CPP is important for sufficient oxygenation of the brain following TBI. However, maintaining a CPP > 70 using fluids and vasopressors has been shown to increase the risk of ARDS. The BTF counsels against induced hypertension as an alternative to reducing ICP. The objective of monitoring is to maintain optimal cerebral perfusion and oxygenation and avoid secondary injury. The recommended means of monitoring ICP is via an intraventricular catheter.

- *Rosen's Emergency Medicine - Concepts and Clinical Practice. 8th edition. 2013. Chapter 41: Head Injury. 356-360.*

- *Brain Trauma Foundation. Guidelines for the Management of Severe Traumatic Brain Injury. 3rd Edition. 2007. full text*

#28

You are seeing a patient in whom you suspect a subdural hemorrhage (SDH). TRUE statements about a SDH include which of the following?

(Choose three answers.)

    A. SDH lies beneath the dura mater, are distributed over the cortex, and appear as a crescent shape.

    B. SDH may extend across suture lines.

    C. SDH can arise from parenchymal bleeding and can be arterial, venous, or from rupture of the bridging cortical veins.

    D. SDH is less common than epidural hemorrhages (EDH).

    E. Mortality of SDH is lower than that of EDH.

#28

Answer: A, B, and C

SDH is much more common than EDH, and it occurs in 12-29% of patients with severe TBI. The midline shift can be larger than the hematoma itself, suggesting underlying brain injury. The brain injury can also result as the hematoma creates direct pressure on adjacent tissue. Because of the associated brain injury, the delay in clinical signs, and the advanced age of the afflicted population, the mortality is much higher than with EDH. Guidelines recommend that acute SDH with either a thickness > 10mm or a midline shift greater than 5mm be evacuated surgically, regardless of the GCS.

- *Rosen's Emergency Medicine - Concepts and Clinical Practice. 8th edition. 2013. Chapter 41: Head Injury. 363-365.*

- *Heegaard W, Biros M. Traumatic brain injury. Emerg Med Clin North Am. 2007; 25(3): 655-78. full text*

#29

You are seeing an elderly patient with a history of atrial fibrillation on warfarin who has had a traumatic head injury with evidence of subarachnoid blood on the head CT. Which of the following has recently become commercially available in the US (previously available in Europe) for the reversal of warfarin in patients with intracranial hemorrhage (ICH)?

A. Vitamin K

B. rFVIIa

C. FFP

D. Prothrombin complex concentrates (PCC)

E. None of the above

#29

Answer: D

PCCs are human plasma derived and undergo viral inactivation. They contain vitamin-K dependent coagulation factors II, VII, IX, and X. Recent evidence suggests that PCCs may be an effective alternative to FFP for the reversal of Coumadin in the acute setting. 4 Factor PCCs have recently become available in the United States under trade name Kcentra.

Using a reversal protocol of 2 units of FFP and 10 mg Vitamin K IV followed by another 2 units of crossmatched FFP, Ivascu, et al. demonstrated decreased time for reversal from 4.3 hours to 1.9 hours, with a subsequent improvement in mortality from 48% to 10%. Alternatives to FFP such as rFVIIa have also been tested.

rVIIa rapidly treats mild to moderate coagulopathy. It decreases time to neurosurgical intervention (144 vs. 446 minutes) and decreases the use of blood products. However it is not considered the standard of care and increases the risk of thrombosis. Other alternatives include vitamin K, PCC, and cryoprecipitate. Note that the administration of vitamin K may not be helpful in the initial immediate reversal, but it may help lessen the rebound effect when the FFP is consumed. Limited evidence shows that subcutaneous administration of vitamin K is inferior to IV and oral administration, which have equivalent efficacy for reversal.

PCC dosing for anticoagulation reversal is 25–50 IU/kg. The 2012 CHEST Antithrombotic Guidelines recommend the use of PCC over FFP for patients with life-threatening bleeds while anti-coagulated on warfarin.

- *Ivascu FA, et al. Rapid warfarin reversal in anticoagulated patients with traumatic intracranial hemorrhage reduces hemorrhage progression and mortality. J Trauma. 2005; 59(5): 1131-7.*

- *Holbrook A, et al. Evidence- based management of anticoagulant therapy: antithrombotic therapy and prevention of thrombosis, 9th ed: American College of Chest Physicians evidence-based clinical practice guidelines. Chest 2012. 141(s2): e152S-e184S. full text*

#30

Which of the following statements are TRUE regarding urethral trauma?

(Choose three answers.)

- A. Urethral injuries are common and most often result from penetrating trauma, such as a gunshot wound, stabbing, or a bite from an animal or human.

- B. Injuries of the urethra are more commonly seen in females.

- C. The male urethra is divided by the urogenital diaphragm into the anterior and posterior division.

- D. The degree of pubic symphysis diastasis and amount of displacement of pubic bone fracture fragments are predictors of urethral injury.

- E. Anterior urethral injuries often result from blunt force trauma to the perineum.

#30

Answer: C, D, and E

Urethral injuries are rare, constituting about 10% of all injuries to the GU system. Urethral injuries are seen almost exclusively in the male population with a higher incidence in males 15-25 years of age. In the female population, urethral injuries almost always occur in relation to pelvic fractures or vaginal laceration. Blunt rather than penetrating trauma is more commonly associated with urethral injuries.

- *Rosen's Emergency Medicine - Concepts and Clinical Practice. 8th edition. 2013. Chapter 47: Genitourinary System. 481-484.*

#31

You are entertaining the diagnosis of a bladder injury in your patient who has a pelvic fracture, and the trauma surgeon asks for a CT cystogram. Which of the following are TRUE statements regarding how this is performed?

A. Retrograde filling of the bladder must be performed with a minimum of 350 ml of contrast material.

B. Post-drainage radiographs needs to be obtained to check for contrast extravasation behind a formally distended bladder.

C. Both of the above are true.

D. Neither of the above is true.

#31

Answer: A

Like plain film cystography, CT cystography is done by performing retrograde filling of the bladder with a minimum of 350 ml of contrast material. Post-drainage images through the decompressed bladder are not necessary since extravasation behind the bladder will be seen on axial sections.

• *Rosen's Emergency Medicine - Concepts and Clinical Practice. 8th edition. 2013. Chapter 47: Genitourinary System. 485-490.*

#32

You are seeing a 21 year old patient who had blunt head trauma with some LOC for 5 seconds during a soccer game yesterday. She was seen in your ED then and had a head CT and blood work, all of which were normal. She now returns with "dizziness" and some headaches, as well as some nausea, but no vomiting. Her exam is completely normal. You should:

    A. Repeat her CT scan.

    B. Perform a CT Angiogram of her brain.

    C. Provide reassurance and remove from play for one more week.

    D. Administer phenytoin.

    E. Administer narcotic agents.

#32

Answer: C

Considerable confusion persists among physicians and the public regarding concussion and the post-concussion syndrome. In general, the degree of amnesia correlates with the duration of loss of consciousness and degree of trauma. Patients can have anterior and retrograde amnesia. The post-concussion syndrome can involve disabling symptoms that consist of recurrent headaches, dizziness, and difficulty concentrating. Data from controlled trials are lacking to guide treatment of the post-concussion syndrome. However, reassurance and education about the effects of concussion have been shown to reduce the incidence and duration of symptoms at 6 months. Patients should avoid narcotics and high doses of NSAIDS which can cause further rebound headaches. Brain rest by avoiding stressful activities and excessive stimulation may offer the greatest benefit.

• Ropper AH, et al. Concussion. N Engl J Med. 2007 Jan 11; 356(2): 166-72. full text

#33

At least how many adjacent ribs must be fractured to be considered a flail chest?

    A. 1

    B. 2

    C. 3

    D. 4

    E. 5

#33

Answer: C

Flail chest results when three or more adjacent ribs are fractured at two points, allowing a freely moving segment of the chest wall to move in paradoxical motion. Because of its common association with pulmonary contusion, it is one of the most serious chest wall injuries.

- *Rosen's Emergency Medicine - Concepts and Clinical Practice. 8th edition. 2013. Chapter 45: Thoracic Trauma. 433.*

#34

The management for flail chest should include all of the following EXCEPT:

(Choose two answers.)

- A. Positioning the patient with injured side down
- B. Placing sandbags on the affected segments
- C. Oxygen
- D. Analgesia
- E. Intensive chest physiotherapy

#34

Answer: A and B

The patient should not be positioned with the injured side down or have weight applied to the affected segments, due to the inhibited expansion of the chest and potential for increase atelectasis of the injured lung.

Oxygen should be administered while the patient is maintained on cardiac monitoring. The most common traumatic complications are pneumothorax and hemothorax, so the patient should be repeatedly reassessed. Also due to pain, there will be incomplete lung expansion and increased risk of atelectasis, requiring physiotherapy and aggressive pain control. If a patient was intubated, the positive pressure ventilation can internally splint the chest wall and make flail segments difficult to detect on initial trauma survey.

- *Rosen's Emergency Medicine - Concepts and Clinical Practice. 8th edition. 2013. Chapter 45: Thoracic Trauma. 434.*

#35

You are seeing a 20 year old male after a high-speed motor vehicle crash. You suspect a diaphragmatic rupture. TRUE statements about this diagnosis include which of the following?

(Choose two answers.)

    A. When diaphragmatic rupture secondary to blunt trauma occurs, the right hemidiaphragm is more commonly affected.

    B. An overlooked diaphragmatic injury in the acute phase sometimes presents as hernia with obstruction, incarceration, or perforation of bowel many years later.

    C. CT of the abdomen and pelvis has a 100% sensitivity and specificity.

    D. Laparoscopy is preferred for the diagnosis and repair of left sided diaphragmatic injury.

    E. All of the above

Amy Kaji

#35

Answer: B and D

If diaphragmatic rupture occurs in blunt trauma, it is more likely on the left side, due to the protective effect of the liver on the right. Chest X-rays are often not diagnostic, and CT scans will be more diagnostic of a left sided injury but have varying reported sensitivities well below 100%. Laparoscopy is the modality of choice for diagnosis and repair of diaphragmatic injuries.

- *Rosen's Emergency Medicine - Concepts and Clinical Practice. 8th edition. 2013. Chapter 45: Thoracic Trauma. 443-444.*

748

#36

You are seeing a patient who complains of the sudden onset of pain, cyanosis, and tenderness of the third toe. True statements about the Blue Toe Syndrome include which of the following?

A. Posterior tibial and dorsalis pedis pulses are typically non-palpable.

B. The septic micro emboli are the most common cause.

C. Involvement is usually bilateral and symmetric.

D. Treatment is directed toward identifying and removing the proximal source of atheroembolism.

#36

Answer: D

Atheroemboli break from proximal atherosclerotic plaques or aneurysms and occlude distal arteries. With the Blue Toe Syndrome, embolic occlusion often presents with a patient complaining of a cool, painful, cyanotic toe in the presence of palpable distal pulses. The occlusion occurs at the level of the microvasculature, not at the level of the dorsalis pedis or posterior tibial artery. Treatment is directed toward identifying and removing the proximal source of atheroembolism and preventing further ischemia with anticoagulation.

- *Rosen's Emergency Medicine - Concepts and Clinical Practice. 8th edition. 2013. Chapter 87: Peripheral Arteriovascular Disease. 1138.*

#37

You are seeing a patient who has a known 4.0 cm aneurysm from a CT scan performed 2 years ago. Unfortunately, he has been lost to follow-up. He complains of back pain and hematuria. His blood pressure is 135/75 and his heart rate is 100. Which of the following should be performed?

(Choose four answers.)

    A. Surgical consultation

    B. Place large bore intravenous lines

    C. Type and crossmatch

    D. Aggressive crystalloid based resuscitation

    E. Radiographic imaging

#37

Answer: A, B, C, and E

An aneurysm producing symptoms should be assumed to be ruptured and expanding until proven otherwise. Even if a patient is hemodynamically stable, they require immediate surgical consult, large bore IV access as well as preparation for potential transfusion with 4-6 units of PRBCs. Aggressive crystalloid based fluid resuscitation should not be started unless there is evidence of peripheral hypoperfusion. Large volumes of crystalloid may dislodge a temporarily stable clot and cause a dilutional coagulopathy.

- *Rosen's Emergency Medicine - Concepts and Clinical Practice. 8th edition. 2013. Chapter 86: Abdominal Aortic Aneurysm. 1133-1137.*

#38

You are seeing a patient who presents with complaints of severe abdominal pain, which is disproportionate to what you find on physical exam. You suspect mesenteric ischemia. Which of the following is the gold standard diagnostic imaging test?

A. Ultrasound

B. Plain radiograph

C. Angiography

D. CT angiography

E. Bedside Laparoscopy

#38

Answer: D

Although angiography was once viewed as the gold standard, it is no longer routinely performed due to its invasiveness and time required. CT angiography (CTA) has replaced it due to the quality of images and speed in the ED. The diagnostic accuracy is high, with a sensitivity of 96% and specificity of 94%. CTA signs confirming the diagnosis can include visualization of the thrombus in the celiac, SMA, and or IMV, venous gas, pneumatosis intestinalis, bowel wall thickening, lack of bowel wall enhancement, and solid organ infarction.

• *Rosen's Emergency Medicine - Concepts and Clinical Practice. 8th edition. 2013. Chapter 95: Disorders of the Large Intestine. 1272-1273.*

#39

You are seeing a patient who was in a motor vehicle accident and are trying to determine if he needs an abdominal CT. In patients with isolated blunt abdominal trauma, which of the following clinical predictors would not allow you to forgo an abdominal CT?

A. Patient has a small apical pneumothorax.

B. Patient has a normal mental status.

C. Patient has a hematocrit of 36%.

D. Patient has no RBCs on urinalysis.

E. Patient has an SBP of 135/75 mmHg.

#39

Answer: A

When evaluating for occult abdominal injury in isolated abdominal trauma, patients can be considered low risk for adverse outcome and may not need abdominal CT scanning if the following are absent:

1. Abdominal tenderness
2. Hypotension
3. Altered mental status (GCS < 14)
4. Costal margin tenderness
5. Abnormal chest radiograph
6. Hematocrit < 30%
7. Hematuria (defined as ≥ 25 RBC/hpf).

• Diercks DB, et al. Clinical Policy: Critical Issues in the Evaluation of Adult Patients Presenting to the ED with Acute Blunt Abdominal Trauma. Ann Emerg Med. 2011; 57: 387-404. full text

#40

You are performing a Focused Assessment with Sonography for Trauma (FAST) examination. A medical student asks you why you are doing this. Which of the following are indications for doing a FAST?

(Choose two answers.)

    A. To determine whether there is intra-abdominal fluid or pericardial fluid

    B. To detect blood in the retroperitoneum

    C. To detect bowel injury

    D. To detect contained solid organ injury

    E. Assessment of penetrating torso trauma to determine if immediate operative management is indicated

#40

Answer: A and E

FAST can be used to assess blunt thoracoabdominal trauma with significant mechanism of injury, but it should never delay a patient's transport to the operative room when operative management is clearly indicated. The ultrasound's sensitivity for retroperitoneal blood, bowel injury, and contained solid organ injury is quite poor. Note that FAST examination may be obscured by obese body habitus, subcutaneous air, pregnancy, pre-existing peritoneal fluid, or increased bowel gas. The inferior pole of both kidneys must be visualized to avoid missing early fluid/blood accumulation. Placing the patient in Trendelenburg position increases the sensitivity of the examination of the right and left upper quadrant.

- *Rosen's Emergency Medicine - Concepts and Clinical Practice. 8th edition. 2013. Chapter 196: Ultrasound. 2494.*

#41

A five-year old boy is accidentally pinned between a car and a garage wall when his father arrives home from work. Regarding his potential injuries, which of the following is TRUE:

A. Pulmonary contusion is very unlikely in children, due to their relatively flexible thoracic cage.

B. Traumatic diaphragmatic hernia, although likely, can be ruled out reasonably with plain chest films.

C. Traumatic asphyxia may be initially apparent only by evidence of physical exam findings such as petechiae or cyanosis above the clavicles.

D. Traumatic aortic disruption can be ruled out with a normal chest X-ray.

#41

Answer C

Traumatic asphyxia results from sudden, massive, direct compression on the chest. It is more common in children due to the compliant chest wall and immature valves of the superior and inferior venae cava. Exhalation against a closed glottis transmits pressure to the heart, lungs, brain, head, and neck, leading to bleeding and/or organ damage. Physical findings include petechiae on the head and neck, subconjunctival hemorrhage, and cyanosis above the clavicles.

Pulmonary contusion is common in children after severe blunt force to the lungs causing parenchymal bleeding. Initial plain films may be normal.

Traumatic diaphragmatic hernia is uncommon in children. It is usually associated with penetrating injuries, often found only during surgical exploration. Chest films will only aid in diagnosis if significant herniation occurs.

Traumatic aortic rupture is rare in children; death most often occurs prior to arrival to the hospital. CT may be used in clinically stable patients with an equivocal chest X-ray or those with negative films but with signs of aortic injury.

- *Rosen's Emergency Medicine - Concepts and Clinical Practice. 8th edition. 2013. Chapter 44: Neck. 430.*

#42

With respect to the adult patient with blunt abdominal trauma, which of the following is TRUE?

(Choose two answers.)

A. In a hemodynamically unstable patient with blunt abdominal trauma, DPL is the diagnostic modality of choice.

B. Oral contrast is not required in the diagnostic imaging for evaluation of blunt abdominal trauma.

C. A clinically stable patient with isolated abdominal trauma (blunt) who has had a negative abdominal CT may be safely discharged.

#42

Answer: B and C

In hemodynamically stable patients with blunt abdominal trauma, bedside ultrasound, can identify patients who require emergent laparotomy. Clinically stable patients with isolated blunt abdominal trauma can be safely discharged after a negative result for abdominal CT with IV contrast. Further observation, close follow-up, and/or imaging may be warranted in selected patients based on clinical judgment.

- *Diercks DB, et al. Clinical Policy: Critical issues in the evaluation of adult patients presenting to the ED with acute blunt abdominal trauma. Ann EmergMed. 2011 Apr; 57(4): 387-404. full text*

UROLOGY

Amy Kaji

#1

Regarding penile disorders, which of the following statements is FALSE?

A. Phimosis is asymptomatic adults can be treated on an elective outpatient basis.

B. Paraphimosis can mimic balanitis unless there is recognition that the foreskin is retracted.

C. Failure to reduce paraphimosis can lead to glans ischemia.

D. When severe phimosis causes urinary retention, a dorsal slit in the foreskin facilitates access to the urethral meatus.

E. A patient with paraphimosis should be referred for 24-48 hour outpatient urology follow-up for reduction.

#1

Answer: E

Paraphimosis occurs when the retracted foreskin is not replaced, usually after cleaning. The constricting foreskin ring then causes edema, venous stasis, and ischemia to the glans. Paraphimosis requires definitive treatment in the emergency department. In contrast, phimosis in asymptomatic patients can be treated on an outpatient basis. However, phimosis can progress to urinary retention if left untreated.

- *Rosen's Emergency Medicine - Concepts and Clinical Practice. 8th edition. 2013. Chapter 99: Selected Urologic Problems. 1349-1350.*

#2

A 17 year old male has an ultrasound that is diagnostic of testicular torsion. The urologist says that he is on his way in, but he asks you to attempt manual detorsion. Which of the following statements is FALSE?

A. Successful manual preoperative detorsion results in a increased testicular salvage rates.

B. Light sedation or spermatic cord block may be done to lessen the patient's discomfort.

C. Most testes twist in a medial-to-lateral direction, so manual detorsion should initially be attempted from lateral to medial, similar to closing a book.

D. One to three turns is usually sufficient, and the detorsion is stopped when the testicular pain is relieved.

E. The patient should still be evaluated by a urologist even if manual detorsion is successful.

#2

Answer: C

Most testes twist in a lateral-to-medial direction, so manual detorsion should initially be attempted from medial to lateral, similar to opening a book. The testis is rotated 180 degrees in one direction and maintained in position. One to three turns is usually sufficient, and the detorsion is stopped when either the anatomy is restored or the testicular pain is relieved. The patient should still be evaluated by a urologist if manual detorsion is successful. Also in cases where there is high suspicion for torsion, a non-confirmatory ultrasound and inability to manually reduce in the ED, urology should still emergently evaluate the patient.

- *Rosen's Emergency Medicine - Concepts and Clinical Practice. 8th edition. 2013. Chapter 99: Selected Urologic Problems. 1343-1346.*

#3

A patient has a staghorn calculus identified on CT scan. Which of the following management strategies is most likely to lead to treatment failure.

    A. Percutaneous nephrolithotomy

    B. Medical management with antibiotics and pain control

    C. Shock wave lithotripsy

    D. Open surgery

    E. Combined nephrolithotomy and shock wave lithotripsy

#3

Answer: B

Staghorn calculi refer to branched stones that fill the renal pelvis and branch into several or all of the calices. The calculi are most often composed of struvite (magnesium ammonium phosphate) and/or calcium carbonate apatite and complicated by urinary tract infections and pyelonephritis. Long term calculi can cause renal failure, and severe sepsis. Surgical removal is the definitive treatment and can be performed via open surgery, percutaneous nephrolithotomy, or shock wave lithotripsy.

- *Rosen's Emergency Medicine - Concepts and Clinical Practice. 8th edition. 2013. Chapter 99: Selected Urologic Problems. 1341-1342.*

#4

Which of the following are the two tests used to confirm the diagnosis of urinary retention?

(Choose two answers.)

A. Urinalysis

B. BUN/Cr

C. Urine Sodium, Osmolality, and Creatinine

D. Post-void residual

E. Ultrasound

#4
Answer: D and E

A post-void residual greater than 100 ml of urine or greater than 20% of voided volume suggests urinary retention. An emergency department ultrasound can document bladder distension suggestive of outlet obstruction, as well. It is important to determine the reason for obstruction and exclude serious neurologic disease such as spinal cord compression. Placing a urinary catheter and decompressing the bladder will quickly relieve the pain. The most common cause is mechanical obstruction in men due to prostatic hypertrophy and medication related causes in women.

- *Rosen's Emergency Medicine - Concepts and Clinical Practice. 8th edition. 2013. Chapter 99: Selected Urologic Problems. 1349-1352.*

#5

Bladder mucosal hemorrhage and post-obstructive diuresis are two complications of bladder decompression, particularly in the patient with chronic urinary retention. Regarding these complications, which of the following is FALSE?

    A. When post-obstructive diuresis of greater than 1 liter per hour occurs, a milliliter for milliliter replacement of the diuresed fluid is indicated.

    B. Bladder mucosal hemorrhage is thought to be the result of sudden expansion of bladder wall veins following decompression.

    C. It is not necessary to clamp the foley catheter to limit the amount of drainage and prevent mucosal hemorrhage.

    D. None of the above statements are false.

#5
Answer: A

It is believed that the large post-diuresis observed after bladder decompression is an appropriate correction of volume overload. Therefore, the milliliter-for-milliliter replacement of this diuresed fluid is not indicated. If the patient becomes hypotensive after foley placement, then fluid replacement should be given. Isotonic saline is usually sufficient with the most common electrolyte abnormality being salt wasting nephropathy. In the past, clamping of the catheter following a certain amount of drainage was recommended in an attempt to avoid bladder mucosal hemorrhage, however this is no longer required.

- *Rosen's Emergency Medicine - Concepts and Clinical Practice. 8th edition. 2013. Chapter 99: Selected Urological Problems. 1351-1352.*

#6

The differential diagnosis of urinary retention in a woman should include all of the following, EXCEPT:

A. Multiple sclerosis

B. Diabetes

C. Hemorrhagic cystitis

D. Calculi

E. Diuretics

#6

Answer: E

Drugs that can lead to urinary retention include alpha adrenergic agents, anticholinergics, antihistamines, opioids, antispasmodics, antidepressants, and antiparkinsonian agents. Diuretics and alpha adrenergic antagonists would contribute to urinary incontinence, not urinary retention. Large bladder calculi or blood clots from hemorrhagic cystitis or cancerous hemorrhage, can all cause obstruction. In women with urinary retention, MS and diabetes should be considered as underlying causes.

- *Rosen's Emergency Medicine - Concepts and Clinical Practice. 8th edition. 2013. Chapter 99: Selected Urologic Problems. 1349-1352.*

#7

Complications of ureteral stents include which of the following:

    A. Infection

    B. Migration

    C. Obstruction from encrustation

    D. All of the above

#7

Answer: D

All three are common complications. If a patient with a ureteral stent manifests symptoms of urinary infection or pyelonephritis, therapy with antibiotics that provide adequate coverage for Pseudomonas should be started promptly. If the patients' anatomy does not allow for perfect alignment of the ureteral stent either in the bladder or the renal pelvis, the stent can migrate either up proximally or distally. Acutely patient's can develop pyelonephritis or obstruction. Chronically, if ureteral stents are not removed or changed in 3 months, patients may develop encrustation around the stent, and hydronephrosis or renal failure can result.

- *Rosen's Emergency Medicine - Concepts and Clinical Practice. 8th edition. 2013. Chapter 99: Selected Urologic Problems. 1341-1342.*

#8

Which of the following is NOT a predisposing risk factor for a perinephric or renal abscess?

    A. Diabetes mellitus

    B. Staghorn calculi

    C. Male gender

    D. Vesicoureteral reflux

    E. Neurogenic bladder

#8

Answer: C

Predisposing factors include diabetes mellitus or a urinary tract abnormality such as an obstructing stone, malignancy, or polycystic kidney. Conditions which cause urinary stasis such as a neurogenic bladder are also implicated. Male gender is not a predisposing risk factor. Renal and perinephric abscess are complications of urinary tract infection that usually occur in the setting of ascending infection with obstructive pyelonephritis (usually due to gram negative enteric bacilli or polymicrobial infection). However, they can also be caused by bacteremia seeding from an alternate source.

- *Rosen's Emergency Medicine - Concepts and Clinical Practice. 8th edition. 2013. Chapter 99: Selected Urologic Problems. 1328-1331.*

Amy Kaji

#9

Risk factors for acute prostatitis include:

    A. Urethral stricture following gonorrhea infection

    B. Trauma

    C. Indwelling bladder catheter

    D. Dehydration

    E. All of the above

#9

Answer: E

All of the above factors have been identified as risk factors for acute prostatitis. The typical signs and symptoms of acute prostatitis include fever, chills, dysuria, pelvic or perineal pain, and cloudy urine. These symptoms are similar to those of a urinary tract infection. Isolated acute cystitis does not commonly occur in men, and many lower UTIs are due to prostatitis. Clinical symptoms together with an edematous and tender prostate on exam should prompt a presumptive diagnosis of acute prostatitis.

- *Rosen's Emergency Medicine - Concepts and Clinical Practice. 8th edition. 2013. Chapter 99: Selected Urologic Problems. 1349-1352.*

#10

All of the following are complications of acute prostatitis EXCEPT:

A. Chronic prostatitis

B. Prostatic abscess

C. Bacteremia

D. Paraphimosis

E. Epididymitis

#10

Answer: D

Complications of prostatitis include bacteremia, epididymitis, chronic bacterial prostatitis, and prostatic abscess. The total duration of antibiotics is for four to six weeks.

Prostatic abscess should be suspected when infection persists despite appropriate antimicrobial therapy. The diagnosis of abscess is made by CT scan. Treatment involves antibiotic targeting gram-negative organisms as well as a urology consult.

- *Rosen's Emergency Medicine - Concepts and Clinical Practice. 8th edition. 2013. Chapter 99: Selected Urologic Problems. 1349-1352.*

#11

Paraphimosis occurs when the foreskin in the uncircumcised male is retracted behind the glans penis, and cannot be returned to its normal position. Regarding paraphimosis, all of the following are true EXCEPT:

A. The constricting foreskin impedes blood flow to the glans and can rapidly progress to distal ischemia.

B. In infants and young children, paraphimosis usually results from self manipulation by the child or inappropriate retraction of the foreskin by the caretaker during cleaning.

C. In the sexually active adolescent or adult male, retraction during intercourse is a potential cause.

D. The majority require emergent urologic consultation for reduction.

E. Iatrogenic paraphimosis follows cystoscopy or bladder catheterization if the foreskin is not reduced back over the glans penis by the medical provider.

#11

Answer: D

Paraphimosis reduction is performed by compressing the swollen glans and the foreskin and slowly withdrawing the foreskin over the glans. Often ice or compression wrapping can decrease edema. The "puncture method" has also been described and requires the use of a 21- to 26-gauge needle to puncture openings into the foreskin to allow edematous fluid to escape from the puncture sites during manual compression.

A dorsal penile block can also be used to reduce pain during the reduction. Patients should also be examined for a concomitant balanoposthitis and referred for elective circumcision after successful reduction in the ED. Only if the reduction is not successful after multiple attempts, is urology consult necessary due to the high risk of ischemia to the glans.

- *Rosen's Emergency Medicine - Concepts and Clinical Practice. 8th edition. 2013. Chapter 99: Selected Urologic Problems. 1349-1350.*

- *Roberts and Hedges' Clinical Procedures in Emergency Medicine. 6th edition. 2013. Chapter 55: Urologic Procedures. 1225-1124.*

Amy Kaji

#12

A 24 year old male presents with scrotal pain and swelling of his left testicle. All of the following findings would lead you to suspect epididymitis, rather than testicular torsion EXCEPT:

A. Normal cremasteric reflex

B. Gradual onset of symptoms

C. Normal to increased testicular blood flow

D. High riding transversely oriented testes

E. Positive Prehn's sign

#12

Answer: D

Most torsions are caused by an underlying anatomic abnormality. Bell-Clapper deformity is due to high attachment of the tunica vaginalis which allows the testicle to freely rotate on the spermatic cord and orients the long axis of the testes in transverse position. Torsion usually begins suddenly and is often associated with nausea and vomiting. It can occur after exertion or during sleep. A normal cremasteric reflex is helpful in excluding torsion except in young children where the reflex may be absent. Prehn's sign is positive when lifting the affected testicle results in symptom relief. This is suggestive of epididymitis. The presence of pyuria, bacteriuria, dysuria or fever does not exclude the diagnosis of torsion. Doppler ultrasonography is useful to verify testicular perfusion. No physical finding is sensitive or specific enough to diagnose the disease and high clinical suspicion is required.

- *Rosen's Emergency Medicine - Concepts and Clinical Practice. 8th edition. 2013. Chapter 99: Selected Urologic Problems. 1342-1349.*

#13
You are seeing a 25 year old female with fever, costover-tebral angle tenderness to palpation and dysuria with suspicion for pyelonephritis. In which of the following scenarios would further imaging be most appropriately indicated?

A. She is a diabetic but is non-toxic appearing, has normal vital signs, and is tolerating oral liquids and solids.

B. She is pregnant 4 weeks by dates.

C. She is sent in from specifically for a CT scan, and she requests one.

D. This is her second visit and she was treated with outpatient ciprofloxacin and she now appears clinically worse.

E. Her father has renal cell carcinoma.

#13

Answer: D

Patients with persistent fever or clinical symptoms after 48 to 72 hours of appropriate antimicrobial therapy for uncomplicated pyelonephritis should undergo radiologic evaluation of the upper urinary tract with ultrasound or computed tomography (CT) scan. The most common complications are an obstructing ureteral stone, abscess, papillary necrosis or emphysematous pyelonephritis.

- *Rosen's Emergency Medicine - Concepts and Clinical Practice. 8th edition. 2013. Chapter 97: Renal Failure. 1306-1307.*

#14

Complicated pyelonephritis is progression of upper urinary tract infection to renal corticomedullary abscess, perinephric abscess, emphysematous pyelonephritis, or papillary necrosis. Risk factors for progression to complicated pyelonephritis include which of the following:

A. Urinary tract obstruction

B. Urologic dysfunction

C. Antibiotic resistant pathogens

D. Diabetes

E. All of the above

#14

Answer: E

Complicated pyelonephritis is progression of the upper urinary tract infection to perinephric abscess, corticomedullary abscess, emphysematous pyelonephritis, or papillary necrosis. In general the major risk factors are antibiotic resistance, diabetes, and obstruction. Diabetes specifically increases the risk for emphysematous pyelonephritis and papillary necrosis. Acute complicated pyelonephritis is associated with pyuria and bacteriuria, although these findings may be absent if the infection does not communicate with the collecting system or if the collecting system is obstructed.

- *Rosen's Emergency Medicine - Concepts and Clinical Practice. 8th edition. 2013. Chapter 97: Renal Failure. 1306-1307.*

#15

You are seeing a 55 year old male with painless hematuria. TRUE statements about painless hematuria include which of the following?

(Choose three answers.)

A. The combination of CT urography and cystoscopy provides optimal evaluation of the urinary tract in a high risk patient for malignancy.

B. Ultrasound provides optimal evaluation of the urinary tract in the high risk patient.

C. Among both men and women, the incidence of malignancy is higher with macroscopic vs. microscopic hematuria.

D. CT urogram is the preferred study for pregnant patients.

E. The risk for malignancy is increased in older individuals (>50yo) who smoke.

#15

Answer: A, C, and E

Painless hematuria is most often benign except in patients over the age of 50 or with a smoking history. The cancers of concern are bladder, renal and prostate. Once active hemorrhage, is excluded, most of the diagnostic evaluation take place as an outpatient. CT urogram (CTU) and cystoscopy will allow for assessment of of the complete genitourinary symptom.

Ultrasonography has a lower diagnostic yield and is less sensitive in detecting urothelial transitional cell carcinoma, renal masses, and calculi. The relative insensitivity of ultrasonography in detecting small renal tumors was shown in a study in which ultrasonography detected only 26% of lesions less than 1 cm and only 60% between 1 and 2 cm. However, with CTU there is a high associated radiation dose. CTU should not be used in pregnant woman.

- *Rosen's Emergency Medicine - Concepts and Clinical Practice. 8th edition. 2013. Chapter 99: Selected Urologic Problems. 1352-1354.*

- *Warshauer DM, et al. Detection of renal masses: sensitivities and specificities of excretory urography/linear tomography, US, and CT. Radiology. 1988 Nov; 169(2): 363-5.*

#16

You are seeing a patient in whom you suspect testicular torsion. Which of the following statements about the diagnosis is TRUE:

(Choose two answers.)

A. The finding of WBCs in the urine definitively excludes the diagnosis of torsion (in favor of epididymitis or orchitis).

B. Manual detorsion should only be performed by the urologist after a confirmatory ultrasound.

C. Salvage of the testicle is nearly 90-100% as long as the testicle is detorsed within 6 hours.

D. The cremasteric reflex may be absent on the affected side.

E. The detection of color or power doppler signal definitively excludes the diagnosis of torsion.

#16

Answer: C and D

Urinalysis results are usually normal. However, the presence of white blood cells (WBCs) can be observed in as many as 30% of patients who have torsion; therefore, WBC presence can not be relied upon to exclude the diagnosis.

Most torsions twist inward and toward the midline; thus, manual detorsion of the testicle involves twisting outward and laterally. It should be performed in the ED prior to ultrasound confirmation. Rotation of the testicle may need to be repeated 2-3 times for complete detorsion and to provide pain relief to the patient. Manual detorsion has success rates that range from 26.5% to 80%.

The detection of color or power Doppler signal in a patient presenting with the clinical findings suggestive of testicular torsion does not absolutely exclude torsion. Clinical correlation should be incorporated in the evaluation of the acute painful scrotum because color Doppler ultrasonography is not 100% sensitive.

A salvage rate of 90-100% is found in patients who undergo detorsion within 6 hours of pain; the viability rate decreases to between 20% and 50% after 12 hours; and 0 to 10% if detorsion is delayed greater than 24 hours. An absent cremasteric reflex is highly suggestive of torsion and its presence may help to distinguish other causes of acute scrotal pain from testicular torsion.

  • *Rosen's Emergency Medicine - Concepts and Clinical Practice. 8th edition. 2013. Chapter 99: Selected Urological Problems. 1343-1345.*

#17

You are seeing a patient with a paraphimosis and have already attempted manual reduction. The urologist on-call asks you to attempt the iced-glove method and the use of babcock clamps. Which of the following are TRUE about these three methods?

A. Analgesia should be used, whether with topical, dorsal nerve, or penile ring block.

B. The iced glove method makes use of ice to provide compression and vasoconstriction.

C. The babcock method requires 6 babcock clamps without serrated edges to evenly and circumferentially grasp the phimotic ring.

D. All of the above

#17

Answer: D

For the iced glove method, a mixture of crushed ice and cold water should be placed in a glove and tied closed at the cuffed end. The thumb of the glove can then be inverted into the glove, thereby producing a condom-like apparatus surrounded by ice water. As much of the penis should then be placed into the thumb of the glove, and the ice and glove will provide compression and vasoconstriction. After about 10 minutes, manual reduction should be attempted.

With the babcock method, six babcock clamps should be placed circumferentially around the phimotic ring. Slow, steady distal traction should be placed on the clamps while using one's thumbs to apply proximal pressure to the glans.

- Houghton GR. The "iced-glove" method of treatment of paraphimosis. Br J Surg. 1973; 60(11): 876-7.

- Skoglund RW Jr, Chapman WH. Reduction of paraphimosis. J Urol. 1970 Jul; 104(1): 137.

#18

You are concerned about a urethral injury in a trauma patient that you are evaluating. He has blood at his urethral meatus and his CT of the abdomen and pelvis demonstrates multiple pelvic fractures. Regarding the retrograde urethrogram which of the following is FALSE?

A. A baseline KUB should be obtained to ensure the film captures the entire course of the urethra and the bladder.

B. The penis should be stretched vertically upward towards the abdominal wall.

C. In an adult 60 ml of water-soluble contrast should be used.

D. 10% water-soluble contrast should be used, and the KUB should be obtained when the last 10 ml of contrast is being infused.

E. You may insert a foley catheter a few centimeters into the urethra when injecting the contrast.

#18

Answer: B

The procedure is performed with the following:

1. Ensure a KUB X-ray can capture the urethra and bladder on a single image
2. Retract the foreskin in uncircumcised patients
3. Stabilize the penis with a 4 by 4 inch gauze
4. Stretch the penis obliquely over the proximal thigh to ensure visualization of the entire urethra.
5. Fill a 60 mL syringe with 10% water-soluble contrast and attach to foley cath or use a plain tip syringe
6. Insert the catheter tip or syringe into the meatus ensuring a tight fit
7. Ensure that there is no contrast leakage during the injection
8. Re-image with a KUB X-ray to assess for extravasation.

A partial disruption is demonstrated by urethral extravasation with contrast entering the bladder. In a complete disruption, no contrast will enter the bladder.

- *Roberts and Hedges' Clinical Procedures in Emergency Medicine. 6th edition. 2013. Chapter 55: Urologic Procedures. 1149-1150.*

#19

Regarding acute urinary retention, which of the following statements is TRUE?

A. The Coudé catheter is frequently necessary to use in pediatric acute urinary retention.

B. The Coudé catheter should be placed with the tip pointing downward to the urethral meatus.

C. Both of the above

D. Neither of the above

#19

Answer: D

Indications and contraindications for use of the Coudé catheter are the same as for foley catheter placement, but the Coudé catheter is usually used after failure of foley placement due to difficult passage. Placing the Coudé is the same as placing a foley except the catheter is placed into the meatus of the penis with the curved tip *pointing up*, dorsally, and is advanced past the resistance point, typically at the level of the prostatic urethra.

The Coudé catheter is rarely used in pediatric patients and should be used cautiously in patients at risk for urethral strictures. One complication is the passage of foley into a false tract if there is a existing urethral injury.

- *Vilke GM, et al. Evaluation and treatment of acute urinary retention. J Emerg Med. 2008 Aug;35(2):193-8. full text*

#20

Which of the following is TRUE regarding performing a dorsal slit procedure?

A. The indication for performing a dorsal slit include inability to void and ischemia to the penile urethra.

B. Relative contraindication to performing a dorsal slit include bleeding dyscrasias.

C. Both of the above

D. Neither of the above

#20

Answer: C

Phimosis with inability to urinate or ischemia to penis is the emergent indication for performing a dorsal slit. Bleeding dyscrasia is the only relative contraindication.

The procedure is performed with the following steps:

1. In a sterile fashion clean and drape the penis
2. Using a 27-gauge needle and lidocaine inject the foreskin on the dorsal aspect proximally to distally.
3. Slide a hemostat along the space between the foreskin and the glans, and gently open, forming a tract.
4. Then, clamp the foreskin with the hemostats with one tip tip between the foreskin and glans, and one tip outside the foreskin. (Avoid the urethral meatus throughout the procedure.)
5. Close the hemostat over the region of anesthesia and clamp for 5 - 10 min.
6. Remove the hemostat, and cut the clamped tissue with iris scissors.
7. Retract the foreskin and clean the glans.
8. Place a foley catheter if the patient has persistent difficulty with urination.

- *Vilke GM, et al. Evaluation and treatment of acute urinary retention. J Emerg Med. 2008 Aug; 35(2):193-8. full text*

#21

The most common causes of urinary obstruction include:

A. Medications

B. Physical obstruction, such as benign prostatic hypertrophy (BPH)

C. Both of the above

D. Neither of the above

#21
Answer: C

Acute obstruction of urinary outflow is most often the result of physical blockages or by urinary retention caused by medications. The most common anatomic cause of obstruction is benign prostatic hypertrophy (BPH) in males and medication (in males or females). Other causes are listed below.

Common Anatomic Causes of Acute Urinary Obstruction

- Benign prostatic hypertrophy
- Prostatic trauma/avulsion
- Bladder calculi
- Prostatitis
- Bladder hematoma/clots
- Urethral inflammation post urethral procedures or manipulation
- Bladder neoplasm
- Urethral strictures or foreign body
- Cystitis
- Phimosis/Paraphimosis
- Meatal stenosis
- Prostate cancer
- Neurogenic etiologies
- Penile trauma

. *Vilke GM, et al. Evaluation and treatment of acute urinary retention. J Emerg Med. 2008 Aug; 35(2):193-8. full text*

#22

Regarding ureteral calculi, which of the following is FALSE?

A. The incidence of kidney stones in the general population appears to be increasing, as does the medical cost associated with this disease.

B. The majority of individuals with urolithiasis have small (<5 mm) stones, located in the distal ureter, that are able to pass spontaneously.

C. Both stone expulsion and time to expulsion of ureteral stones depend heavily on stone size and location.

D. Urologic intervention is recommended for ureteral stones that persist for more than 2 months.

E. A meta-analysis demonstrated that neither calcium channel blockers nor alpha-antagonists increase the rate of stone passage.

#22

Answer: E

A pooled analysis of 16 studies using an α-antagonist and 9 studies using a calcium channel blockers suggested a benefit to these therapies when compared to standard therapy, in terms of improved stone expulsion in patients with distal ureteral stones.

- α-antagonist RR 1.59; 95% CI 1.44 to 1.75; NNT 3.3 [95% CI 2.1 to 4.5]
- calcium channel blocker RR 1.50; 95% CI 1.34 to 1.68; NNT 3.9 [95% CI 3.2 to 4.6]

Adverse effects were noted in 4% of patients receiving α-antagonist and in 15.2% of patients receiving calcium channel blockers.

The authors conclude from this meta-analysis that there is a significant benefit in the stone expulsion rate when either an α-antagonist or calcium channel blocker is added to standard therapy in the medical management of moderately sized distal ureteral stones. However, small stones, which are less than 5 mm, will likely pass regardless of medical therapy.

Although meta-analyses of previous randomized controlled trials concluded that the smooth muscle relaxant drugs tamsulosin and nifedipine assisted stone passage for people managed expectantly for ureteric colic, a randomized placebo-controlled trial demonstrated that no difference was noted between active treatment and placebo (p=0.78), or between tamsulosin and nifedipine (p=0.77).

- *Singh A, et al. A systematic review of medical therapy to facilitate the passage of ureteral calculi. Annals of Emerg Med. 2007; 552-563. full text*

- *Pickard, R et al. Medical expulsive therapy in adults with ureteric*

Amy Kaji

colic: a multicentre, randomised, placebo-controlled trial. 2015; epub.
full text

#23

TRUE statements about bladder stones include which of the following?

   A. Bladder stones constitute a different entity from that of renal stones.

   B. The most common cause of bladder stones is infection of residual bladder urine with urea-splitting organisms.

   C. Plain radiographs of the pelvis reveal a bladder stone in 50% of cases.

   D. All of the above

#23

Answer: D

Although calculi generally form in the kidneys, they also may originate in the bladder. Bladder stones differ from renal stones since they occur almost exclusively in elderly men. Most bladder stones are caused by urea-splitting organism such as Proteus or from chronic indwelling catheters and urinary stasis. Bladder outflow obstructions, neurogenic bladder, vesical diverticula, radiation and schistosomiasis are other causes. The stones can cause sudden and intermittent cessation of urination as the stone obstructs the bladder outlet. Plain radiographs are diagnostic in 50% of cases. Depending on the size, the stones may pass spontaneously or require surgical intervention.

- *Rosen's Emergency Medicine - Concepts and Clinical Practice. 8th edition. 2013. Chapter 99: Selected Urological Problems. 1342.*

#24

You are seeing a 45 yo male in whom you suspect a varicocele causing the appearance of a scrotal mass. TRUE statements about varicoceles include which of the following?

(Choose two answers.)

    A. These are more common on the right side.

    B. Most varicoceles are asymptomatic.

    C. Varicoceles are usually more symptomatic when standing and relieved when laying flat.

#24

Answer: B and C

Varicoceles are enlarged spermatic cord veins. A varicocele, can either be idiopathic or the first sign of a retroperitoneal tumor, renal cell carcinoma, or renal vein thrombosis. The left side predominates because the left testicular vein drains perpendicularly into the left renal vein, while the right testicular vein drains obliquely into the inferior vena cava. Patients are usually only symptomatic upon standing or during activities that increase intra-abdominal pressure. In most cases, outpatient urologic followup is sufficient.

• *Rosen's Emergency Medicine - Concepts and Clinical Practice. 8th edition. 2013. Chapter 99: Selected Urological Problems. 1349.*

www.ingramcontent.com/pod-product-compliance
Lightning Source LLC
Chambersburg PA
CBHW052306220526
45472CB00001B/2